MW01688146

TIMES AND TIDES OF TUBERCULOSIS

Medical History Books by Thomas M. Daniel

Polio
(editor, with Frederick C. Robbins)

Captain of Death: The Story of Tuberculosis

Pioneers of Medicine and Their Impact on Tuberculosis

Drama and Discovery. The Story of Histoplasmosis
(with Gerald L. Baum)

Wade Hampton Frost. Pioneer Epidemiologist. 1880–1938. Up to the Mountain.

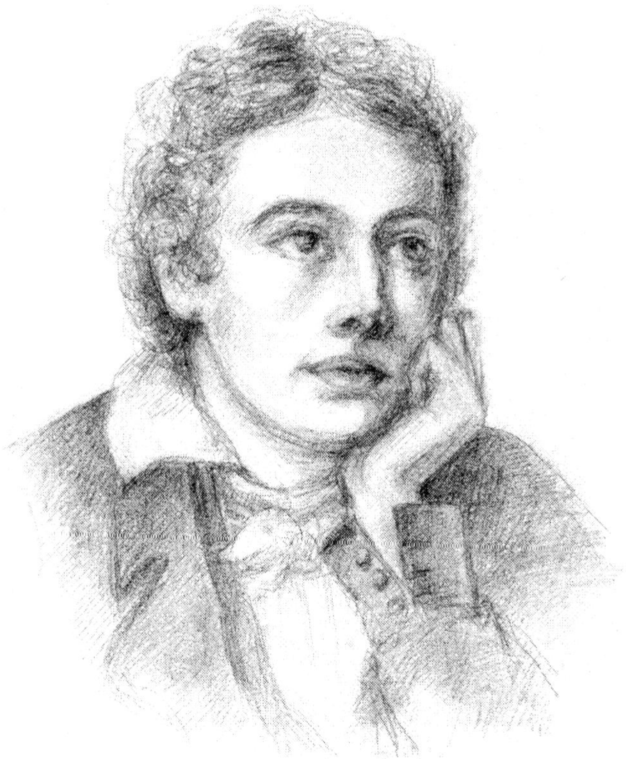

JOHN KEATS, 1795-1821
Pencil drawing by Shannon Casey

TIMES AND TIDES OF TUBERCULOSIS

Perceptions Revealed in Literature, Keats to Sontag

Thomas M. Daniel

2013 · FITHIAN PRESS, MCKINLEYVILLE CALIFORNIA

Cover photograph by Arthur B. McComb, May 3, 1988.
Abandoned building of the White Haven Sanatorium. The White Haven Sanatorium opened in 1901 and operated until it closed on March 1, 1956. It housed an average of 617 tuberculosis patients annually. It attempted to provide free or low-cost care for tuberculosis victims of limited means.

Published by Fithian Press
A division of Daniel and Daniel, Publishers, Inc.
Post Office Box 2790
McKinleyville, CA 95519
www.danielpublishing.com

Distributed by SCB Distributors (800) 729-6423

LIBRARY OF CONGRESS CATALOGING-IN-PUBLICATION DATA
Daniel, Thomas M., 1928- author.
Times and tides of tuberculosis : perceptions revealed in literature, Keats to Sontag / by Thomas M. Daniel.
pages cm
ISBN 978-1-56474-544-6 (pbk. : alk. paper)
1. Tuberculosis in literature. 2. Literature and medicine—History.
3. Tuberculosis—History. 4. Diseases in literature. I. Title.
PN56.T82D36 2013
809'.933561—dc23
2013005476

For Janet

Who loves me, helps me, and encourages me.
Without her this book would not have been possible.

Pray, of what disease did Mr. Badman die? For I now perceive we are come up to his death.

I cannot so properly say that he died of one disease, for there were many that had consented, and laid their heads together, to bring him to his end. He was dropsical, he was consumptive, he was surfeited, was gouty, and, as some say, he had a tang of the foul distemper in his bowels. Yet the captain of all these men of death that came against him to take him away was the consumption, for it was that that brought him down to the grave.

—John Bunyan
The Life and Death of Mr. Badman

Diseases manifest multiple personalities just as do living creatures and social institutions. The various moods which they display in different circumstances and at any given time reflect the dominant aspect of the relationship between the disease process and the life of man in society.

— René and Jean Dubos
The White Plague: Tuberculosis, Man, and Society

CONTENTS

PREFACE

THIS BOOK is about tuberculosis. It is not, however, a text. It says little about the etiology or pathogenesis of tuberculosis, nor the signs and symptoms of the clinical illness. I have written about those and other features of the disease in texts, scientific reviews, and research reports.

This is a book about history. It presents two centuries of the history of tuberculosis. Yet it does not recount the global spread of that disease. Nor does it chronicle tuberculosis from its ancient origins in Africa. I have written about those aspects of the disease in books, chapters, and articles.

This is a book about books. And about poetry and short stories and journals and letters written by authors. It is a book rooted in literature. This book examines attitudes towards and perceptions of tuberculosis. It does so by considering descriptions of tuberculosis and its victims in words written by those affected by the disease. It examines changes in those attitudes over time as reflected in those writings over time.

Tuberculosis was the focal point of my professional career. I witnessed much of the evolution of the drug treatment of tuberculosis. Inevitably, my background and professional experience with the disease have influenced this book in what I hope is a positive fashion.

As I thought about the many richly written descriptions of the disease, I decided to base this work on published literature. There is much to choose from, and I chose works that illustrate the range of views for each of three epochs—no available treatment, sanatorium care, and curative drug therapy.

As I have presented the works of individual authors selected for inclusion in this book, I have tried to set the times and life circumstances of those writers. I have told the stories of their lives briefly. I have told the stories of their encounters with tuberculosis in more detail. I have quoted from their works and their letters to reveal their attitudes towards tuberculosis. Insight into literature is gained from understanding the circumstances of its creation.

I have read and reread the works quoted in this book. While I have focused on the authors' perceptions of tuberculosis, I have also offered interpretations of their works. Good literature does more than tell a simple story. There are evocative images, metaphors, and symbolisms included that convey ideas and concepts. Thus, I have provided interpretations, and they are solely mine. Although I have consulted the many, usually scholarly works of critics in this regard, I have relied on my personal understanding of what the chosen authors wished to communicate.

This is a carefully researched work. Yet I have tried to avoid pedantry. One does not need to be a phthisiologist (tuberculosis expert) to enjoy this book. One does not need to be a historian nor a literary critic. Tuberculosis affected and continues to affect ordinary people. Ordinary people are and long have been interested in tuberculosis. Ordinary people can gain insights into tuberculosis from the words of talented writers.

ACKNOWLEDGMENTS

"WHERE DID you find those quotes?" asked a friend who had just read an early draft of one of this book's chapters.

"I read the book," I replied, somewhat testily.

This work depends upon and derives from published literature. My own personal library contains many of the works cited; I pulled from its shelf my copy of the source of the quotation queried by my friend. Other works came from public and university libraries. I owe much to the libraries and librarians of Case Western Reserve University in Cleveland, Ohio, where I am an emeritus professor of medicine and international health. The Kelvin Smith Library contains a rich trove of classic literature and biographies of noted authors. I spent hours seated at cubicle desks in the Kelvin Smith stacks. Librarians and many work-study students helped me find volumes that seemed in hiding, especially including librarian Janet Klein. I used the copy machines in the library, and I used my faculty card to check out individual volumes.

Many people have been helpful to me in writing this book. I particularly want to thank Roger Allen for ferreting out information about Derek Lindsay; Martha Brandt Pollock for helpful insights into Henry David Thoreau; Ted and Felicia Justin for driving me to Haworth and the Brontë Museum in Yorkshire on two occasions; Hannah Scanlon for comments on the professional tennis world of Alice Marble; Leslie Sowle for insightful comments on the works of the Brontë sisters; and Ned Yost and Tim Marrs for helping in my attempt to sort out the meaning of Mann's Hofrat.

My younger brother, John, an author, editor, and publisher, gave me much helpful advice as I navigated my route from laboratory bench to word processor.

Above all others, I am grateful to my wife, Janet, who has read and helped edit every page of this book through multiple revisions.

TIMES AND TIDES
OF TUBERCULOSIS

INTRODUCTION

Over the course of human history tuberculosis has afflicted and killed hundreds of millions of people. It was carried across the globe by early humans as they migrated from Africa, and evidence of it exists worldwide in early archeological sites. Slowly mounting to reach epidemic proportions in Europe, this flood of disease peaked in the early nineteenth century. We do not have accurate statistics based on case reporting for that era, but 1819, when John Keats developed tuberculosis, is a reasonable choice for a starting point in the narrative, and the one used in this book. Our story begins then. At that time tuberculosis may have been responsible for as many as one in four deaths in Europe. Since then, the tide of this disease has slowly ebbed. Today it is known to most persons in the medically advanced world as a malady that may have shown up in a grandparent or other forebear but is of no current concern.

The history of the great epidemic of tuberculosis can be divided into three time periods. At the time of its peak and during most of the nineteenth century, it was a disease evoking despair. Physicians could offer nostrums relieving some symptoms, but no meaningful solace. With the discovery of the cause of tuberculosis and the openings of sanatoria devoted to its treatment at the end of the nineteenth century, there was some hope for improvement, if not complete recovery. The advent of curative drugs in the mid-twentieth century ushered in an era of cure and expectations of recovery. This era with its expectation of the recovery of health and well-being dates to a series of drug discoveries in the latter half of the twentieth century. They began in 1944, with the discovery of streptomycin and continue to the present.

Tuberculosis remains with us today, however, especially in Sub-Saharan Africa and Southeast Asia. More than a million people die of this disease each year. It is worth recalling its history and the threat that any resurgence would impose.

One can recount the history of tuberculosis in many ways. This book does so in the words of a series of persons who suffered from the disease. They were not ordinary people, however. They were authors whose writings reflect their experience with the dread disease. They were intelligent people, generally well-educated among their peers, and their words were written with skill. We can only assume that those with the talent and inspiration to put pen to paper reflected the views of other, less literary people. What they wrote was widely read and enjoyed at the time; what they wrote remains readable and enjoyable today.

To provide context for the literary excerpts used to illustrate the impact of tuberculosis on its victims, Part I of this book describes the historical period covered by the work. In this single-chapter section, the changing times and evolving knowledge of disease are briefly recounted. Modalities of treatment shifted with the emergence of theories and knowledge of the life-threatening disease. As they changed, so also did the expectations of afflicted persons.

The subsequent Parts II, III, and IV of this book present the lives and writings of authors afflicted by tuberculosis in its three time periods, each characterized by distinct prospects for those suffering from the disease. A final coda in Part V notes that the threat of this disease remains with us and recounts the challenges presented in seeking new means of addressing the threats of the Captain of Death.

PART I

EBB AND FLOW

—The Changing Tides of the White Plague—

CHAPTER 1

CHANGE

What then should be our strategy,... if we are to treat and prevent all of these infectious diseases?

—Richard M. Krause, The Restless Tide: The Persistent Challenge of the Microbial World.

IN 1819 a well-dressed young woman wore linen drawers and a crinoline petticoat under her flowing skirt. In 1978 she wore cotton bikini briefs under her tight jeans. In 1819 a traveler crossed the Atlantic Ocean in several weeks on a sailing ship. In 1978 a traveler crossed the Atlantic in several hours in a jet engine-powered aircraft flying several miles above the sea.

In 1819 John Keats developed tuberculosis. In the same year René Théophile Hyacinthe Laennec published his work, *De l'auscultation médiate* that unified the concept of tuberculosis as a single disease. In 1978 Susan Sontag published *Illness as Metaphor,* in which she noted that earlier attitudes towards tuberculosis had been shifted to cancer. In that year curative drug treatment of tuberculosis was widely available.

Over the course of sixteen decades the way people in the western world lived changed dramatically. Over those same decades the impact of tuberculosis on people's lives changed, and so also did their perceptions of the disease. Knowledge of the disease and treatment of it also evolved.

In the early nineteenth century an epidemic of tuberculosis raged. René and Jean Dubos, both sufferers from the disease themselves, called it the "White Plague," thus distinguishing its slow but inexorable spread from the tsunami-like onslaught of bubonic plague, the

"Black Death," which killed one-fourth to one-third of the residents of European cities in the fifteenth century. Just when the surging tide of tuberculosis peaked in Europe and North America is not knowable; the late eighteenth century is a reasonable surmise. The tuberculosis death rate in England in 1780 has been estimated at an astonishing 1,120 deaths per 100,000 population per year. The tide was almost certainly ebbing during the nineteenth century. One should not suppose that it was no longer a major problem, however. At the Hôpital de la Charité in Paris, one in three deaths in the early nineteenth century were due to tuberculosis. It may have caused one fourth of all deaths in Europe in 1815. In London the death rate was falling, but it was still 567 deaths per 100,000 per year in the early 1830s. The peak of the tuberculosis epidemic arrived somewhat later in North America than it did in Europe. In the mid-nineteenth century, urban American death rates approximated 400 per 100,000 per year; they fell slowly thereafter.

Charles Dickens was a prolific and popular novelist of the nineteenth century, and for the most part he focused on the lives of those downtrodden by the events and circumstances of the times. *The Life and Adventures of Nicholas Nickleby* was first published serially, as were many novels of that time, between April 1838 and October 1839. Nicholas Nickleby, Dickens's protagonist, befriends a much-abused young boy named Smike, with whom he escapes from a tyrannical schoolmaster to join a traveling troop of actors. Smike suffers from tuberculosis. Writing sentences in his characteristic style, with its seemingly verbose pedantry; writing with redundancies—needless, perhaps, but expressive—and with punctuation which, to the modern reader, perhaps, seems quixotic, even illogical; writing in sentences that seem at times interminable, but are yet expressive—sentences carefully crafted; writing words to be read in leisurely fashion, words that are both expressive and descriptive, words to be savored; writing for a readership that prized detailed description; Dickens describes Smike's illness in the following sentence:

> There is a dread disease which so prepares its victim, as it were, for death; which so refines its grosser aspect, and

> throws around familiar looks, unearthly indications of the coming change; a dread disease, in which the struggle between soul and body is so gradual, quiet, and solemn, and the result so sure, that day by day, and grain by grain, the mortal part wastes and withers away, so that the spirit grows light and sanguine with its lightening load, and, feeling immortality at hand, deems it but a new term of mortal life; a disease in which death and life are so strangely blended, that death takes the glow and hue of life, and life the gaunt and grisly form of death; a disease which medicine never cured, wealth never warded off, or poverty could boast exemption from; which sometimes moves in giant strides, and sometimes at a tardy sluggish pace, but, slow or quick, is ever sure and certain.[1]

Ever sure and certain, death comes to Smike somewhat more than one hundred pages further into the narrative. Dickens describes it as peaceful and a release:

> And now Nicholas began to see that hope was gone, and that, upon the partner of his poverty, and the sharer of his better fortune, the world was closing fast. There was little pain, little uneasiness, but there was no rallying, no effort, no struggle for life. He was worn and wasted to the last degree; his voice had sunk so low, that he could scarce be heard to speak; Nature was thoroughly exhausted, and he had laid him down to die.
>
> On a fine mild autumn day, when all was tranquil and at peace; when the soft sweet air crept in at the open window of the quiet room, and not a sound was heard but the gentle rustling of the leaves; Nicholas sat in his old place by the bedside, and knew that the time was nearly come....
>
> While he was thus employed, the closed eyes opened, and on the pale face there came a placid smile.
>
> "That is well!" said Nicholas. "The sleep has done you good."

> "I have had such pleasant dreams," was the answer. "Such pleasant, happy dreams!"
>
> "Of what?" said Nicholas.
>
> The dying boy turned towards him, and putting his arm about his neck, made answer, "I shall soon be there!..."
>
> He fell into a light slumber, and waking smiled as before; then, spoke of beautiful gardens, which he said stretched out before him, and were filled with figures of men, women, and many children, all with light upon their faces; then, whispered that it was Eden—and so he died.[2]

These two passages, in which Dickens describes Smike's death from tuberculosis, epitomize nineteenth-century attitudes towards this Captain of Death. Inescapable, hopeless, yet somehow gentle. Dreaded, yet accepted. Bringing deliverance from pain. Romanticized.

The medical history of tuberculosis in the nineteenth century had its origins in the work of René Théophile Hyacinthe Laennec. Laennec was born on February 17, 1771 in the Brittany town of Quimper. Following the death of his mother from tuberculosis when he was five years old, he was cared for by relatives, and in 1788 he was sent to live with an uncle, Guillaume Laennec, a surgeon, in Nantes. In Nantes the young Laennec witnessed the horrors of the French revolution; a guillotine was set up opposite his uncle's house. In 1785 he began the study of medicine in Nantes. Laennec then enrolled with Napoleon's army as a surgeon; in those tumultuous times he opposed the revolution, and later he would become a royalist. In 1801 Laennec went to Paris, where he enrolled in the École de Médecine at the Hôpital de la Charité. There he and his friends and colleagues, Marie François Xavier Bichat and Gaspard Laurent Bayle, studied with France's leading physician, Jean Nicolas Corvisart. Both Bichat and Bayle would soon succumb to tuberculosis. Laennec would outlive them, only to die of the disease later.

In 1804, shortly before he received his degree in medicine, Laennec described his experience with 400 autopsies of people who had died of tuberculosis. In this lecture he presented a unified concept of tuberculosis with its hallmark granulomatous lesions in whatever tissues of the body it might involve. In so doing, he broke with his predecessors who believed that *phthisis* was tuberculosis of the lungs and a distinct and separate disease from tuberculosis in other organs. This presentation marked the beginning of a new understanding of the disease that ranked among the commonest causes of death for centuries. It made tuberculosis one disease, one killer upon which doctors and their patients could focus in the hopes of new understanding and new modalities of treatment. Following Laennec's lead, *phthisis* became a term reserved for tuberculosis of the lungs. Consumption became the name usually given to disseminated tuberculosis.

Laennec became increasingly prominent and respected in the French medical community. His royalist sympathies and devout Catholicism distanced him from the main stream of Parisian medicine, however. When, in 1816, he was awarded a professorial chair, it was not at the central and prestigious Hôpital de la Charité but at the outlying Hôpital Necker. There he continued his autopsy studies of tuberculosis. In 1816 he invented the stethoscope, an instrument that permitted the first effective examination of diseased lungs during life. Its utility was recognized promptly, and physicians flocked to his wards to learn how to use this new diagnostic tool.

Political considerations once again impeded Laennec's career and delayed the publication of his researches. He compiled an authoritative text on the pathology and physical examination signs of tuberculosis titled *De l'auscultation médiate*, which finally appeared in print in 1819. An English version, reorganized and heavily edited by John Forbes, appeared in 1821 with the title *A Treatise on the Disease of the Chest*. Even to the modern reader, this work is remarkable and stands as an elegant exposition of the nature of tuberculous disease.

Throughout his adolescent and adult life, tuberculosis stalked Laennec. During his adult years he became increasingly disabled by pulmonary insufficiency. Beginning in 1818 he spent much of his time in his beloved Brittany, where he felt the clean, ocean air made him better. He built a home in Ploaré on the coast not far from Quimper. He died there on August 13, 1826, a victim of the disease to which he had devoted his career.

Sir James Clark was one of England's most distinguished physicians of the era. He served as physician to Prince Leopold and the Duchess of Kent. Queen Victoria appointed him to her court as Physician in Ordinary and granted him a baronetcy. He lived in Italy for several years, and while there he attended poet John Keats during his final illness.

Clark was born in Scotland in 1788 and originally studied law. He then pursued training in medicine, and in 1809 he became a member of the College of Surgeons of Edinburgh. He served as a naval surgeon with arctic explorer William Parry. Returning to Edinburgh, he pursued further medical studies, receiving an additional degree from Edinburgh in 1817. Tuberculosis soon became the principal focus of his practice. In 1835 he published *A Treatise on Pulmonary Consumption,* which set out in detail his thoughts on the treatment of patients with tuberculosis. In this text Clark estimates that tuberculosis of the lungs caused about one fifth of deaths in Europe and North America. If all forms of tuberculous disease were to be included and infant mortality excluded, then adult mortality from tuberculosis would reach one in three. Clark advocates study of the cause of tuberculosis, and he believes that further understanding of the disease might lead to effective therapy.

> If the labour and ingenuity which have been misapplied in fruitless attempts to cure an irremediable condition of the lungs, had been rightly directed to the investigation of the causes and nature of tuberculous disease, the subject of our inquiry would have been regarded in a very different light from that in which it is at the present period.
>
> By a knowledge of the causes of the morbid condition of the system in which tuberculous disease had its origin, we may reasonably hope to prevent the occurrence of the latter in many cases, and in a small proportion to arrest its progress.[3]

Clark discusses the treatment of tuberculosis. The measures he recommends are palliative—intended to bring relief and comfort, if not healing and an unattainable cure. Travel and a move to a benign climate were recommended by many physicians of the era, and Clark espouses this approach. "Travelling is attended with many advantages. Independent of its physical effects, the change of scene and the constant succession of new objects exert a direct and most beneficial influence."[4]

Blood letting had become a widely used form of treatment of tuberculosis, especially when the patient experienced hemoptysis (coughing of blood). Phlebotomy (literally, opening a hole in a vein) probably had its origin as a measure to remove evil humors thought to be causing disease. When the patient was seen to be expelling humor-bearing blood by coughing, it would then be logical to remove more blood. Clark attributes the introduction of this practice into Britain to Thomas Dovar, who published a tract advocating its vigorous use in 1733. Dovar bled his patients for six to eight ounces of blood at a time! Clark, ever mindful of the comfort of his patients, does not reject bleeding, but he argues for restraint. "The employment of general bloodletting...requires, in my opinion, great judgment and circumspection. The more general error is the abstraction of too great a quantity of blood at a time."[5]

Clark favors some of the local remedies then in common use. He considers cupping—the application to the skin of a heated cup or wine glass which, when it cooled, would exert suction—to be "very beneficial" when applied to the upper chest. He also accepts the use of leeches—a method of removing blood commonly enough used so that physicians of the era were colloquially called "leeches"—but cautions against their "too free application." He argues in favor of the daily use of skin irritants, such as camphor and turpentine, while regulating their use according to the sensitivity of the skin and discomfort they cause. Throughout Clark's text, he makes a point of considering the comfort of his patients.

The first half of the nineteenth century surely was a time when tuberculosis was a dread disease. Both sufferers and those who cared for them knew that hope was beyond hope for those afflicted with tuberculosis. One must accept the inevitable fate of those stricken by the dread disease.

The end of the nineteenth century, a century of misery, brought changes that offered eagerly received hope to the victims of tuberculosis. New understanding of the disease and new approaches to its treatment ignited sparks of optimism.

Jean-Antoine Villemin was a French army surgeon. Born on a farm in the Vosges Mountain of Eastern France on January 25, 1827, Villemin joined the army and began training in military medicine in 1849. Two years later he joined the faculty of the Val-de-Grâce military medical college, then located in Strasbourg and later in Nancy, where he remained for the rest of his career. He became interested in tuberculosis, and was given a small, rudimentary laboratory, where he began studies of this disease. In 1865 he first demonstrated the transmissible nature of tuberculosis.

> [On] March 6, 1865, we took two rabbits about three weeks old [and] very healthy. In one of these rabbits we introduced into a little subcutaneous wound behind each ear, two small fragments of tubercle and a small amount of purulent liquid from a tuberculous cavity...of a consumptive who had been dead twenty-three hours.... At the end of three months and fourteen days, there was no appreciable change in the health of the animal,...[and so] we sacrificed it.[6]

When the tissues of the sacrificed rabbit were examined, tuberculous lesions were found to be widely disseminated in the animal. The uninfected rabbit was free of disease. That the diseased animal was apparently healthy despite the multiple lesions reflects the fact that rabbits are not generally susceptible to tuberculous infection, even when widespread; had he done his experiments with guinea pigs, he might have observed an even more dramatic outcome. Villemin repeated his experiment with additional animals, and his work was slowly recognized. He was honored by election to the French Academy of Medicine in 1867. He died in 1892 at the age of sixty-five.

Heinrich Hermann Robert Koch was born on December 11, 1843 in the Harz Mountain village of Clausthal. After studying medicine at Göttingen, where he was exposed to some of the leading medical scientists of the time, he became District Medical Officer in Wollstein, Silesia (now the Polish city of Wolsztyn). There he provided medical care to the community. His mind reached beyond the duties of his post, however, and he soon began investigating anthrax, a serious local problem. With encouragement from his wife, he set up a laboratory and darkroom in his home. Soon he had worked out the life cycle of the spore-forming bacterium that causes anthrax and had taken history's first photomicrographs of bacteria to document his findings.

Koch showed his work to the eminent pioneer of bacteriology, Ferdinand Cohn, who found a position in Berlin for the remarkable young physician. In Berlin Koch set to work to determine the cause of tuberculosis, and within an extraordinarily short six months he had identified the tubercle bacillus and proved that it was the cause of tuberculosis. On March 24, 1882, Koch presented his findings to a stunned audience at the Berlin Physiological Society. Fulfilling what are now known as the Koch or Koch-Henle postulates, he had isolated tubercle bacilli in pure culture from diseased persons, had reproduced the disease by injecting the cultured bacilli into guinea pigs, and had once more cultured tubercle bacilli from the diseased animals. Koch's work was immediately acclaimed. He became a medical hero, a hero of unprecedented magnitude. Later Koch repeated his remarkable work of discovery by adding identification of the cause of cholera to those of anthrax and tuberculosis.

Koch always referred to the bacterium he discovered as the tubercle bacillus. Later generations of microbiologists would give it its scientific name, *Mycobacterium tuberculosis*, often abbreviated as *M. tuberculosis*. It is often called, "Koch's bacillus."

Koch's accomplishments cannot be undervalued. Yet, he himself did much to damage his reputation when, in 1891, he announced that he had found a cure for tuberculosis. The product he touted was tuberculin, the forerunner of the material used today for tuberculin skin testing. It did not benefit those who suffered from tuberculosis;

indeed, it made some of them sicker. Soon this remedy was discredited. Koch's reputation recovered, however, and he was awarded the Nobel Prize in Medicine or Physiology in 1905.

With the transmission of tuberculosis and its bacteriological cause now understood, the world believed that medical science and the doctors who practiced medicine would soon be able to alleviate the suffering of the victims of Koch's bacillus. There was reason for hope. The world was ready to welcome new approaches to tuberculosis therapy.

Treatment of tuberculosis during this era of change often meant withdrawal from one's usual life and retreat to a healing place or to a specialized sanatorium. The father of the sanatorium treatment of tuberculosis was Gustav Hermann Brehmer. His ideas about the causes of tuberculosis and its treatment altered the management of the disease for more than one hundred years. On the centenary of Brehmer's birth, S. Adolphus Knopf, a leading tuberculosis specialist of his time, described him as "the great pioneer of modern sanatorium treatment...who has given the inspiration to hundreds, if not thousands, of men to establish sanatoria for the treatment of the tuberculous."[7]

Brehmer was born in Kurtsch in Silesian Prussia on August 4, 1826. He attended the university in Breslau, where he studied natural history and mathematics. He also studied in Berlin, and while there he heard lectures by physiologist Johannes Müller. Inspired by that experience, he completed medical education in Berlin. He then returned to Silesia where he opened a medical practice in Görbersdorf in 1854. His sister-in-law operated a spa specializing in hydrotherapy in Görbersdorf.

Every physician in the nineteenth century treated tuberculosis. Brehmer, however, diverged from usual medical thinking with regard to his patients. He felt that he understood what made people susceptible to tuberculosis and that this understanding logically dictated certain aspects of treatment. Brehmer knew that some cattle taken to graze in high mountain meadows in the summer were found to have enlarged hearts when they were butchered. He did not understand brisket disease, the cause of the ailing and abnormally enlarged hearts in the cattle. However, Brehmer knew that many patients who died of tuberculosis were found at autopsy to have small hearts. He concluded that small hearts made persons susceptible to tuberculosis. In fact, this decrease in heart size was a consequence of the advanced disease, which Brehmer seemed not to recognize. By moving to high altitudes, he reasoned, his patients' hearts—like those of cattle—would enlarge, and thus, he supposed, their resistance to the disease would be amplified.

Brehmer conceived of a spa at Görbersdorf in the Silesian Mountains. More than that, however, Brehmer planned to provide not only the benefits of high altitude but active treatment. For this treatment he embraced the hydrotherapy practiced at his sister-in-law's spa. Central to this treatment were brief daily showers with cold water, and it was important that the physician supervise and regulate every aspect and detail of this therapy.

> The water of douches must be cold and fall with considerable force. The stream must form an even, homogeneous column which should have the same diameter above and below.... The douche is also of particular value for pleuritic exudates, which are very quickly absorbed under its influence. It is, however, a dangerous remedy and should be administered only by the physician.[8]

He prescribed not only cold-water douches, but also a rich diet with wine and daily evening cognac. Hungarian wine was best, because of its high phosphate, lime, and magnesium contents. He promoted physical exercise and brisk outdoor hikes in the mountain air. Activity must also be regulated by the physician, he believed, and he prescribed it with careful consideration of the atmospheric conditions of each day. He built a meteorological observatory to measure wind, humidity, and temperature to aid in formulating his daily activity prescriptions.

Brehmer opened his *Heilanstalt* in Görbersdorf as a small *kurhaus* in 1859. After several expansions, it grew to more than 300 beds in an imposing building, and by 1904 it was the world's largest facility devoted to the treatment of tuberculosis. It is generally considered the first tuberculosis sanatorium. In 1867, Peter Detweiler, Brehmer's disciple, established a sanatorium in nearby Falkenstein. Detweiler disagreed with many of Brehmer's concepts, including his ideas about heart size, and he advocated open air and rest in reclining chairs for his patients. During ensuing decades hundreds of institutions opened for the care of persons with tuberculosis—many in mountainous areas, including four others in Görbersdorf. Davos in the Swiss Alps became a famous haven for consumptives, as did places in the American Appalachian, Adirondack, and Rocky Mountains. Colorado Springs was promoted by real estate developers as a location benefitting those with tuberculosis.

Brehmer's *Heilanstalt* was not the first medical facility dedicated to the care of tuberculosis patients. A Hospital for Consumption and Diseases of the Chest was opened in London in 1841, undergoing several changes over the next few years and ultimately establishing its presence in Brompton in 1849. Today "The Brompton" continues as a premier academic medical center focused on cardiovascular and pulmonary diseases.

In what was certainly one of history's most bizarre attempts to establish a healing place for tuberculosis patients, Dr. John Crogan took sixteen patients deep into Mammoth Cave, Kentucky in 1842. He had purchased the cave in 1839 and built small huts in the cave. One of his patients left after a short time. Five died of tuberculosis while living in the cave. The remaining ten persisted in the subterranean world for a year before struggling out to the surface.

In a church basement on Channing Street in Boston, Harriet Ryan Albee began caring for indigent victims of tuberculosis in 1857; two years later her facility moved to larger quarters and assumed the name of the Channing Home, reflecting its origin. Albee died there of tuberculosis in 1873. It moved into the neighborhood of the Harvard Medical School in 1907.

The first American tuberculosis sanatorium in the model of those of Brehmer and Detweiler was opened in 1875 in the Appalachian Mountains near Asheville, North Carolina, by Joseph Gleitsman. Edward Livingston Trudeau's Adirondack Cottage Sanitarium followed in 1884. Trudeau stressed rest and "the outdoor life" in his management of consumptives. Sanatorium care became the norm for the treatment of tuberculosis. The 1907 *British Journal of Tuberculosis* editorializes:

> Fads and fancies have gathered about so-called "open-air" treatment, and impossible claims have been made by inexperienced enthusiasts as to the almost miraculous efficacy accruing from sanatorium residence. In spite of all exaggerations and failures, there can be no doubt but that [sanatorium care]...offers the best means known to modern medical science for dealing effectively with tuberculosis.[9]

By 1953, as this era of tuberculosis treatment peaked before its abrupt end, there were 839 sanatoria operating in the United States, comprising more than 130,000 beds.

As the nineteenth century passed into the twentieth, a new era for those afflicted with tuberculosis dawned. Sanatoria offered a new approach to the dread disease. Moreover, if sufferers adhered to prescribed regimens and treatments for tuberculosis, there might be reason for hope. They were sure of that, for their doctors told them so. As a consequence of new treatment modes, attitudes towards tuberculosis by its victims and by the general public changed profoundly. Patients arrived at sanatoria with the expectation of improvement, perhaps cure. Indeed, the time spent at these institutions was spoken of as "curing."

Christy Mathewson may have been the best baseball pitcher ever to mount the mound. From the time of his boyhood in Factoryville, Pennsylvania, he displayed enormous pitching talent. In 1901 he joined the New York Giants. He won the first eight games he pitched for the team, three of them as shut-outs. By the end of the season he had pitched in 38 games, 36 of them for the entire game. He won twenty games that year and had an earned run average of 1.99. The ensuing years brought one amazingly successful season after another.

In 1919 Mathewson performed poorly. Some thought he might be throwing games. It soon became apparent that he was ill, and the following year found him at Saranac Lake. His course was a complicated and difficult one, and the "Captain of Death" would ultimately take him. Yet he had hope.

> In baseball we learn to obey orders and follow the rules. We try to make the plays that give us the most chance to win.... I try to keep cheerful, keep my mind busy, try not to worry and I won't change anything.
>
> A fellow begins to feel that life is worth fighting for and to realize something of what it means to lose it. Oddly, a fellow thinks less and less of himself and more and more of others. He has less dread of death.[10]

Today we expect that antibiotics and other drugs will cure most infectious diseases, including tuberculosis. The origins of this expectation are rooted in the mind of Paul Ehrlich. On March 24, 1882, Ehrlich was twenty-five years old, four years out of medical school, and a physician at the Charité Hospital in Berlin when he attended Koch's exposition on the tubercle bacillus and demonstration that it was the cause of tuberculosis. He commented later, "I hold that evening to be the most important experience of my scientific life."[11] While a student Ehrlich had studied organic chemistry and had performed experiments with aniline dyes. With his knowledge of colorants, he set about improving on the techniques Koch used to stain tubercle bacilli, soon developing the methods that underlie those used in microbiology laboratories today. Five years later he was to use his techniques to make his own diagnosis of tuberculosis.

Ehrlich's thinking was rooted in the remarkable specificity of dyes that might stain a microorganism while not staining the surrounding tissues. He worked in the laboratory of Emil von Behring, who developed antiserum for the treatment of diphtheria, and in this work he recognized the great specificity of antibody-mediated reactions. From this he developed a theory of antibody specificity for which he received the Nobel Prize in Medicine or Physiology in 1908. While he missed the mark with many aspects of antibody specificity, his thinking led him to postulate specific receptors. In his Nobel lecture he posited chemical groupings on the molecules of toxins to which antibodies bound, calling them "receptors." It was not then a large leap to think of what he called "magic bullets," drugs that might specifically attack receptors on pathogenic microorganisms. He pursued this line of research, ultimately developing arsenic compounds, arsphenamine and neoarsphenamine, for the treatment of trypanosomiasis in cattle and syphilis in humans, the first specific chemotherapeutic agents for treating infectious diseases. Later mercury replaced arsenic as the standard agent for treating syphilis. Much more important than Ehrlich's contribution to the treatment of syphilis was his concept of specific receptors. It became and remains the basis for the targeting of pharmacologic agents for the treatment of disease.

If arsenic and mercury could benefit infectious diseases, then surely gold must also. It is difficult to believe that this line of thinking had a base in logic rather than alchemy, but it was pursued. Sodium gold thiocyanate, a salt of the precious element, came into use for the treatment of tuberculosis in Denmark in the early 1920s. It was given the drug name of sanocrysin. Its use spread, accepted without data to support its claimed efficacy. In 1926 and 1927 J. Burns Amberson, B.T. McMahon, and Max Pinner conducted a careful study of sanocrysin in tuberculosis patients at the Maybury Sanatorium in Northville, Michigan.[12] These investigators selected twenty-four patients who "were free from severe constitutional symptoms and most of whom had been in the sanatorium for some time and were ambulant.... The pulmonary tuberculous lesions were of the [type described] in the literature [for which] better results are to be expected." By the toss of a coin, half of the patients were assigned to receive injections of sanocrysin and half to receive placebo saline injections. Only the ward nurse who gave the injections and two investigators who were not involved in the care of the patients knew to which group each patient belonged. Careful follow-up revealed that none of the patients given sanocrysin benefitted from it and that many suffered severe liver toxicity. Sanocrysin was ineffective and toxic. Its use was quickly abandoned as the results of this study became known.

The sanocrysin study is important not only because of its impact on an ineffective form of treatment but also because it introduced a method of clinical study. It was the first randomized, placebo-controlled, blinded study in clinical medicine. This method of study was subsequently used for the evaluation of other forms of treatment of tuberculosis, most notably streptomycin. It is now the "gold standard" technique for the evaluation of all forms of pharmacological interventions, including cancer chemotherapy.

Gerhard Domagk was born in 1895 in Lagow, Brandenburg, in what was then eastern Germany, a part of Poland after World War I. He was a university student embarked on a course in medicine in Kiel when war erupted in Europe in 1914. Domagk enlisted in the German army, saw infantry combat service, and was wounded. After the war he returned to complete his medical studies in Kiel. Thereafter he took a position in a pathology institute in Greifswald where he studied the mechanisms by which streptococci produce disease. In 1925 he was appointed to a professorship at the University of Münster. He also began working with two dye chemists, Joseph Klarer and Fritz Meitzsch, at Farbenfabriken Bayer, where he became head of a department of experimental pathology in 1927. The chemists synthesized Prontosil, a red dye, in 1932.

In the laboratory, Prontosil impeded the growth of streptococci. Domagk proceeded to test it in mice, rats, and cats infected with streptococci, and found that it cured these experimental infections and was well tolerated by the animals. Not until three years later did he publish his results. Further study demonstrated that Prontosil was converted to sulfanilamide in the body and that the sulfa compound was the active anti-infective agent. Sulfanilamide had been discovered and patented in 1909 and could not be re-patented. Tentative use in humans with streptococcal infections followed; Domagk's daughter was among the persons treated early. Women with infections relating to obstetrical delivery were treated with success, and in 1939 a child with meningitis was cured. Soon sulfa drugs were the mainstay of treatment of infections due to streptococcal and staphylococcal bacteria. Winston Churchill flew to Tunis to meet General Dwight Eisenhower in December 1943. On the journey there, he contracted pneumonia. He was treated with one of the new sulfa drugs and recovered from what in that day was an often fatal illness.

In 1939 the Nobel Prize committee awarded the Nobel Prize in Medicine or Physiology to Domagk, but the Nazi German government refused to allow him to travel to neutral Stockholm to accept the prize; in 1947 he finally received the Nobel medal.

Sulfa drugs had no effect when tested against tubercle bacilli growing in cultures. The chemists at Bayer continued their work synthesizing various other compounds, and Domagk tested them. A class of agents known as thiosemicarbazones was promising, and Domagk, working through the war years in facilities battered by Allied bombing, found that one later named thioacetazone was effective in halting the growth of *Mycobacterium tuberculosis* (bacteriostatic). As drug regimens were developed, it came into use combined with other agents. Its low cost made it attractive for use in third-world settings.

Acetyl-salicylic acid, commonly known as aspirin, was among chemical compounds studied as it became apparent that some could serve as drugs for fighting infections. Salicylates are good pain and fever relievers. In one form or another, they are the active ingredients of many herbal remedies, and they are the basis for commonly used lineaments. In 1940 Frederick Bernheim at Duke University in North Carolina published a short note in *Science*, the widely-read weekly journal of the American Association for the Advancement of Science, in which he reported that salicylates increased the uptake of oxygen by growing tubercle bacilli.[13] Bernheim's paper was noted by Danish physician Jürgen Lehmann, then working in Stockholm. Working with Swedish chemist colleagues, he soon discovered that para-aminosalicylic acid (PAS), another salicylate, was bacteriostatic for *M. tuberculosis*. Chemists at Ferrosan, a Swedish pharmaceutical company, synthesized the drug. In 1946 Lehmann reported the treatment of twenty tuberculosis patients with PAS in 1944. PAS came into wide-spread use as a second drug combined with other bactericidal agents. It required a dose of twelve grams—typically twenty-four tablets—each day, and was irritating to the stomach. Its first clinical use preceded that of streptomycin by eight months, and

Lehman reacted bitterly to the award of the Nobel prize to Waksman for his discovery of streptomycin.

In the history of the medical conquest of tuberculosis, there are few stories as important or as adorned with as much controversy as that of the discovery of streptomycin, the first agent found to kill *Mycobacterium tuberculosis* (bactericidal). The central figure in this tale was Selman Waksman. Born in the Ukrainian village of Priluka in 1888, Waksman emigrated to the United States in 1910. Accepted into medical school at Columbia University, he found the cost beyond his means, and so he entered Rutgers University, where he studied soil microbiology with Jacob Lipman. He devoted his life to research on soil microorganisms called actinomycetes, organisms he believed to be important to the fertility of humus. In 1916 in the course of his studies of soil actinomycetes while still a student in Lipman's laboratory, Waksman and fellow student Roland Curtis described an organism they named *Actinomyces griseus*, a name later changed to *Streptomyces griseus*. When it became evident that actinomycetes produced antibiotics, the search for more of these disease-fighting drugs became Waksman's central focus.

In 1943 Albert Schatz, a Rutgers graduate student, joined the workers in Waksman's laboratory. In order that he might become familiar with and proficient in the techniques then in use in the laboratory, he was assigned to work with technician Elizabeth Bugie and given the task of characterizing and studying for antibiotic production an organism found in the throat of a sick chicken recently brought to the laboratory. The organism proved to be *S. griseus*, the actinomycete first identified twenty-seven years previously by Waksman and Curtis. Schatz was a prodigious worker, and within two months had isolated the antibiotic that became known as streptomycin. It was effective in killing many microorganisms, including *M. tuberculosis*. Waksman received the Nobel Prize in Medicine or Physiology for the discovery of streptomycin in 1952. The Nobel committee did not include Schatz in the award, a fact that ultimately led to controversy and much bitterness, including a law suit by Schatz.

At the Mayo Clinic in Rochester, Minnesota, Drs. William Feldman and Corwin Hinshaw were studying a number of drugs putatively effective against tuberculosis in guinea pigs infected with tubercle bacilli. They read the reports of Schatz and Waksman, and in November of 1943 Feldman visited Waksman in his Rutgers laboratory. After learning of the work at the Mayo Clinic, Waksman provided Feldman and Hinshaw with a small supply of streptomycin isolated in his laboratory. Used in guinea pigs, it was dramatically effective and nontoxic. Encouraged, they turned to their clinical colleagues and treated a courageous nineteen-year-old young woman whom they felt was likely to die despite receiving rest and a thoracoplasty (a surgical procedure collapsing and putting at rest portions of a diseased lung) at the Mineral Springs Sanatorium in Cannon Falls, Minnesota. Although the initial streptomycin preparations were crude and caused considerable fever and pain, a later supply from Waksman was purer and better tolerated. The young woman improved dramatically, underwent further thoracoplasty, and was discharged to be married and become the mother of three children. Streptomycin was put into production by Merck and Company, and within two years became widely available. Citing the importance of the drug in relieving human suffering, Merck did not seek patent protection for its technology.

Streptomycin proved to be toxic to both the kidneys and the eighth cranial nerve, the nerve serving both the hearing and balance functions of the inner ear. In practice, most patients could tolerate a total of forty grams, almost none eighty grams. Initially given daily in one-gram doses, streptomycin later was given twice weekly when used in multidrug combinations. Streptomycin had to be given by injection, which limited its usefulness as treatment for tuberculosis shifted from hospital to ambulatory settings.

The discovery of isonicotinic acid hydrazide (isoniazid, INH) marked a major turning point in the treatment of tuberculosis. A bactericidal drug not effective against other bacteria, it has proven to be the linchpin for most modern tuberculosis treatment regimens. It was identified independently between 1950 and 1952 in three pharmaceutical industry laboratories, those of Hoffman La Roche, Squibb, and Bayer. Its discovery came as a result of systematic searches among chemicals related to thiosemicarbazones, the drugs studied by Domagk. Because it had been described in published literature many years earlier, it could not be patented. To illustrate the effort put into these searches, scientists at Lederle Laboratories screened "some two to three thousand chemicals against the tubercle bacillus" in a chick embryo system, selecting fifteen percent of them for screening in mice. Although they found some with activity, they failed to include INH in their investigation.

Clinical studies of INH were undertaken soon after its identification. The first to be reported was initiated at Sea View Hospital on Staten Island, one of the boroughs of New York City, on June 19, 1951. Isoniazid and its isomer, iproniazid, were studied in 175 patients with extensive, active pulmonary tuberculosis. The results were first presented to the annual meeting of the American Medical Association on June 10, 1952 and published in the journal of that association on November 8, 1952.[14] Seldom has a drug entered into medicine's therapeutic armamentarium as rapidly and as dramatically. Fever and cough disappeared in all those given one of the drugs. Weight gain was dramatic. Well-being returned, and patients were soon out of bed. *Life* and the *Saturday Evening Post* magazines ran feature articles with photographs of Sea View patients celebrating and dancing and clearly on the road to recovery. Toxicity was minimal for isoniazid; iproniazid was soon abandoned because of its liver toxicity. Modern treatment of tuberculosis with expectation of cure was born with the introduction of isoniazid. All modern treatment regimens include isoniazid in combination with other drugs.

The same search that identified isoniazid yielded pyrazinamide, which is bactericidal (kills bacteria) when used in the initial treatment of tuberculosis. Originally considered too toxic when compared with isoniazid, it later found a place at a lower dose in multidrug regimens.

In 1957 scientists at Lepetit Laboratories in Italy isolated a crude substance from *Streptomyces mediterranei*, subsequently reclassified and renamed *Nocardia mediterranei*, which had antibiotic activity. They called it rifamycin, a name puckishly chosen from the title of a then-popular French movie, *Rififi*. Many years of work followed.

In 1965 rifampin (rifampicin in Europe) was synthesized from a derivative of the parent rifamycin. An agreement was worked out with the Swiss pharmaceutical company, Ciba-Geigy, to produce the new drug. Clinical trials followed and demonstrated it to be an effective bactericidal agent. Rifampin was approved for use in Italy in 1968; the United States Food and Drug Administration approved it in 1971. It was heralded in a March 1969 editorial in the *New England Journal of Medicine* and noted to have engendered excitement "unequaled since the introduction of isoniazid."[15] Rifampin now stands as a major component of all drug regimens for the treatment of tuberculosis and is, perhaps, the single most effective drug available for treating this disease.

The search for additional drugs continued. Many agents effective against other microbial invaders were tested. In the early 1990s a group of compounds known as quinolones emerged as antimicrobial agents. However, their story is actually more than 350 years old. In 1638 Sra. Ana de Osorio, wife of the Spanish viceroy in Peru, was cured of malaria when she was given the bark of the cinchona tree. Returning to Spain three years later, she brought word of this miraculous therapy. Her story intrigued Jesuit Father Joseph Rompel, an Austrian professor of botany, who championed use of the bark. It was imported to Europe and North America, where it became known as the Jesuit bark, and was used to treat many febrile illnesses. Over-harvesting led to the loss of Peruvian sources of the bark, but smuggled seedlings had been planted in Southeast Asia, which then became the world's source for the curative bark. In 1820 the active ingredient of the bark was isolated and named quinine. Quinine remained the standard treatment for malaria until World War II, when Japanese control of the South Pacific prompted a major effort at synthesizing related compounds, including chloroquine, which soon replaced quinine for the treatment of malaria.

The first quinolones were identified as by-products of the synthesis of chloroquine. In the 1990s and early 2000s scientists at pharmaceutical companies began adding fluoride ions to these compounds. The resulting drugs, known as fluoroquinolones, proved to be remarkably effective in the treatment of many infections. Moreover, they proved to be effective against *M. tuberculosis* and rapidly assumed a major place in the treatment of tuberculosis.

A number of other drugs are effective in the treatment of tuberculosis, but none rank with INH, rifampin, pyrazinamide, and the fluoroquinolones. For the most part these other drugs, usually termed "second-line drugs," are used in retreatment of difficult cases, especially when disease is caused by drug-resistant bacilli. Ethambutol, a bacteriostatic drug developed by Eli Lilly and Company in 1963, has been widely used as a companion drug with INH, rifampin, and pyrazinamide in multidrug regimens. Streptomycin has almost entirely dropped out of usage because it has to be given by injection.

The advent of effective drug treatment for tuberculosis heralded the demise of sanatoria. Trudeau's sanatorium in Saranac Lake closed at the end of 1954 for lack of patients. Others followed, sometimes reluctantly as they were firmly entrenched in the medical care system of the era. In 1992 there were only four tuberculosis hospitals with 420 beds in America. Today only one remains, the National Jewish Health Service in Colorado. It specializes in treating drug-resistant disease considered beyond their capabilities by local health departments.

—

Perhaps as a result in part of improved tuberculosis treatment and increased public health efforts, tuberculosis case rates in the western world have plummeted. It is no longer a common disease. Perhaps this decline is simply the usual cycle of most infectious disease epidemics, albeit on a much protracted time line. Tuberculosis now afflicts only about 10,000 Americans each year. Only about 500 Americans die of the dread disease each year. The history of tuberculosis has changed dramatically.

Kevin Patterson titled his 2007 novel *Consumption*. The book chronicles the passing of traditional Inuit life as the modern ways of urban life creep into a small Hudson Bay community. The story begins when tuberculosis strikes six-year-old Victoria. She is sent south to spend the next ten years recovering from the disease. She improves with modern drug therapy, but a large cavity remains. She undergoes a thoracotomy to remove the infected lung lobe and a thoracoplasty to reshape her chest to fit the now reduced lung. Finally well, she returns to her Inuit community, a lovely, mature woman with a deformed body, fluent in French and English but barely able to understand her native tongue, more comfortable in the Hudson Bay Store than her parents' home.

Victoria's tuberculosis serves as a metaphor for the story that unfolds. Snowmobiles and Weetabix replace dog sleds and dried char. The Inuits have no choice but to submit. They survive, but their culture is deformed. They are no longer the people they were and will never again be.

Change is inevitable. One must learn to adapt to it.

Unlike that of Victoria, the lives of most persons living in the western world are not affected by the dread disease. And those whom it does touch now have little to dread.

PART II

HIGH TIDE

—*Captain of Death*—

CHAPTER 2

ROMANTIC POET

JOHN KEATS, 1795–1821

—*Submission*—

Youth grows pale and spectre thin and dies.
—*John Keats,* Ode to a Nightingale

JOHN KEATS was born into a family of modest but comfortable means on October 31, 1795, in Moorfields on the outskirts of London—now engulfed by the spread of the urban metropolis. Nothing in his early life would have suggested that he would one day rank as one of the English language's finest romantic poets. His parents, Thomas and Frances Jennings Keats, operated a livery stables, the Swan and Hoop, originally owned by her parents, who also owned a neighboring pub of the same name. John was the eldest of four surviving children of the couple; he had two brothers, George and Tom, and a sister, Frances, the youngest. Little is known of Keats's genealogic lineage. His father came from Cornwall or Devon and found employment at the Swan and Hoop, where he proved to be able and was made manager. The Keats parents were not highly educated, and there are no literary antecedents in either family.

On the night of April 15, 1804, when Keats was eight years old, his thirty-year-old father fell against an iron railing when his horse stumbled. Newspaper reports at the time indicated that he may have been inebriated. He fractured his skull in the fall and died within hours. Less than three months later, on June 27, Frances married William Rawlings, a bank clerk. That marriage did not last long, and when Frances left Rawlings, her mother, Alice Jennings, took primary responsibility for the care the children.

Keats and his brother George attended the school of John Clark at Enfield, not far from his grandmother's home. He was an average student. Much liked by his fellow students, he was also impetuous and sometimes short tempered. He was schooled in and enjoyed the Greek mythology that was to feature so prominently in his later poetry. It was at Enfield that he met Charles Severn, who would become a successful painter and portraitist and a life-long close friend. Charles Cowden Clarke, son of the schoolmaster and four years older than Keats, also became a good friend.

Despite separation from her maternal care, Keats remained devoted to his mother. She had suffered with arthritis for some time and became seriously ill in December 1809, probably suffering from tuberculosis. The fourteen-year-old Keats took on the responsibility of much of her care, cooking for her, feeding her, and administering medicines to her. Within three months she was dead. Alice Jennings, Keats's grandmother, then moved to establish a guardianship for the Keats children, choosing as trustees John Nowland Sandell and Richard Abbey, a tea dealer. Sandell died two years later, and the further care and financial well-being of the Keats children rested solely with Abbey. There should have been adequate fiscal resources from the Jennings estate to provide each of the children with a modest income, but money was never forthcoming from Abbey. Keats spent much of his life in debt and begging his friends for funds.

In the summer of 1811, Abbey arranged for Keats, then fifteen years old, to be apprenticed to Thomas Hammond, a local surgeon and apothecary. Such an apprenticeship was the usual route of entry into a medical career, and there is reason to believe that Keats looked forward with pleasure to such a prospect. Keats moved into Hammond's house and followed him on his daily rounds, acquiring the surgical skills of dressing wounds, pulling teeth, setting broken bones, and other practical skills of a nineteenth-century physician. Continuing the customary course of medical training of the time, Keats entered the medical school at Guy's Hospital in London, then and today one of Britain's most distinguished medical schools, on October 1, 1815. There he embarked upon a year of medical lectures and anatomical dissections under the tutelage of some of England's preeminent practitioners. He was apparently a good student, and he passed the qualifying apothecary examination on his first attempt in July 1816. At Guy's Hospital, Keats secured an appointment as a dresser, a position somewhat analogous to that of a modern-day hospital intern, which carried with it a salary. This appointment continued until March 1817.

During his later years as a medical apprentice and student, Keats began writing poetry with increasing commitment to this muse. At some time in 1817 he confronted Abbey with his decision to abandon medicine for the life of a poet. Abbey, a man of business, was not sympathetic to this decision, and this added further to Keats's financial straits. But Abbey's disapproval did little to dissuade Keats. Among his notable early works was "On First Looking into Chapman's Homer." He started work on his allegorical, lyric, poetic retelling of the Greek tale "Endymion." Keats's famous opening line, "A thing of beauty is a joy forever," was originally written as "A thing of beauty is a constant joy" during a chemistry lecture. Yet Keats did not regret his study of medicine. In a May 3, 1818 letter to his friend and fellow poet, John Hamilton Reynolds, he wrote:

> Were I to study physic or rather Medicine again, I feel it would not make the least difference in my Poetry; when the Mind is in its infancy a Bias is in reality a Bias, but when we have acquired more strength, a Bias becomes no Bias. Every department of Knowledge we see excellent and calculated towards a great whole. I am so convinced of this, that I am glad at not having given away my medical Books.[1]

As early as some time in 1816, Keats's friend Charles Cowden Clarke showed some of his poems to Leigh Hunt, an influential political rebel, minor poet, and publisher of the liberal journal *The Examiner*. Keats had little interest in politics—his mind was consumed with images of beauty and Greek mythology. An excerpt from "Ode on a Grecian Urn," written in the spring of 1819, epitomizes these facets of Keats's thinking and poetry.

O Attic shape! Fair attitude! With brede
Of marble men and maidens overwrought,
With forest branches and the trodden weed;
Thou, silent form, dost tease us out of thought
As doth eternity: Cold Pastoral!
When old age shall this generation waste,
Thou shalt remain, in midst of other woe
Than ours, a friend to man, to whom thou say'st,
"Beauty is truth, truth beauty,"—that is all
Ye know on earth, and all ye need to know.[2]

Keats was soon drawn into Hunt's circle of radical thinkers, sometimes called "the rascals." It was there he met Percy Bysshe Shelley, whose reputation was somewhat more firmly established than that of Keats. Neither young poet had yet achieved the recognition that would later be accorded to them; Wordsworth and Coleridge were the iconic poets of that time. Initially Shelley and Keats were not friends. In fact, at that time Shelley disparaged Keats's work. Later he would much admire Keats's poetry. Hunt's sponsorship helped launch Keats into a world of poetry, even while it also attached to him an undeserved and inappropriate political aura. It was through Hunt that Keats met Charles Armitage Brown, who would become his close friend.

In early 1818 it became apparent that Tom, Keats's brother, was ill, probably with tuberculosis, and the two brothers went to the Devon coast at Teignmouth, hoping that the sea air would foster a recovery for Tom. Indeed, Tom did improve, but dreary, rainy weather soon convinced them to abandon the shore and return to London. The rain did, however, provide ample time for Keats to retreat to seclusion and complete "Endymion."

Tom's health waxed and waned. He had several episodes of hemoptysis (coughing of blood). On reaching London, he seemed in much better health, and Keats determined to set off on a long-planned and much-delayed walking tour with Charles Brown. They walked through the Lake District and across Scotland to Inverness. They climbed Ben Lomond. During the trip, Keats was recurrently plagued with a sore throat, the cause of which is not clear. After consulting a local physician about his throat, Keats decided to return to London by ship. On return in August, he found his brother to be much worse, and much of his time and effort during the next three months was devoted to caring for his dying brother. Tuberculosis claimed the life of Tom Keats on December 1, 1818; he was nineteen years old.

Following his brother's death on December 18, 1818, Keats moved in with Charles Brown. Brown lived in one of two adjacent rented houses at Wentworth Place. The other house was occupied by the Brawne family. Frances Brawne, Fanny, then age eighteen, caught the eye of John Keats. They were soon in love, and on Christmas Day, 1819, they announced to Fanny's widowed mother their intent to marry. The months of late 1818 and early 1819 were among Keats's happiest and most productive; a number of his poetic works were published and well received.

On February 3, 1820, Keats had his first episode of hemoptysis, and he made his own diagnosis of tuberculosis. His friend, Charles Brown, described the events in the following, often-quoted passage from his early biography of the poet.

> One night, at eleven o'clock, he [Keats] came into the house in a state that looked like fearful fierce intoxication. Such a state in him, I knew, was impossible; it therefore was the more fearful. I asked hurriedly, "What is the matter,—you are fevered?" "Yes, yes," he answered, "I was on the outside of the stage this bitter day till I was severely chilled,—but now I don't feel it. Fevered!—of course, a little." He mildly and instantly yielded, a property in his nature towards any friend, to my request that he should go to bed. I followed with the best immediate remedy in my power. I entered his chamber as he leapt into bed. On entering the cold sheets, before his head was on the pillow, he slightly coughed, and I heard him say,—"That is blood from my mouth." I went towards him; he was examining a single drop of blood upon the sheet. "Bring me the candle, Brown; and let me see this

> blood." After regarding it steadfastly, he looked up in my face, with a calmness of countenance that I can never forget, and said,—"I know the colour of that blood;—it is arterial blood;—I cannot be deceived in that colour;—that drop of blood is my death-warrant;—I must die." I ran for a surgeon; my friend was bled; and, at five in the morning, I left him after he had been, some time, in a quiet sleep.[3]

Keats was seen promptly by the local physician summoned by Brown. He withdrew blood from a vein, a standard form of therapy at that time intended to remove disease-causing humors from the circulation. Keats was confined to bed in a room with all windows closed, as fresh air was thought to be deleterious to health. Later, he was seen by Robert Bree, a specialist in chest diseases, who recommended continuation of the regimen of enforced confinement, bed rest, and bleedings. Keats also took calomel, a mercury-containing medication frequently used for patients with tuberculosis at that time. Keats poured out his soul in daily love letters to Fanny Brawne. Periods of improvement alternated with further progression of his illness.

Physician biographer Walter A. Wells believes that Keats's illness began earlier. He believes that Keats's fatigue during his 1818 walk with Brown and the symptoms for which he consulted a doctor in Inverness, Scotland, were manifestations of pulmonary tuberculosis.[4] Wells's hypothesis is reasonable, for hemoptysis rarely marks the actual onset of tuberculosis; it usually requires well established disease with lung cavities. Ultimately Keats determined that he must go to Italy, where the favorable climate might prove salubrious.

When Shelley learned that Keats had developed tuberculosis with a major hemoptysis, he wrote to Keats on July 27, 1820, urging the ailing poet to come to Italy and stay with him in Pisa.

> My Dear Keats,
> I hear with great pain the dangerous accident that you have undergone, and Mr. Gisborne who gives me the account of it, adds that you continue to wear a consumptive appear-

> ance. This consumption is a disease particularly fond of people who write such good verses as you have done, and with the assistance of an English winter it can often indulge its selection;—I do not think that young and amiable poets are at all bound to gratify its taste; they have entered into no bond with the Muses to that effect. But seriously (for I am joking on what I am very anxious about) I think you would do well to pass the winter after so tremendous an accident, in Italy, and if you think it as necessary as I do so long as you could [find] Pisa or its neighbourhood agreeable to you, Mrs. Shelley unites with myself in urging the request, that you would take up your residence with us.[5]

Keats was determined to go to Rome. He planned to put himself under the care of Dr. James Clark, a distinguished British physician and tuberculosis specialist then in Rome. (Dr. Clark is discussed in Chapter One.) He did not want to spend this time of illness in the free-love ménage that Shelley had established there with his wife, Mary Wollstonecraft, and her sister, Claire. In fact, Keats and Shelley had not been close friends. Keats, for his part, considered Shelley overbearing and found himself uncomfortable with a man of an obviously different social class. John Keats was a man from a middle-class background and a practical person who found it hard to relate both to Shelley's aristocratic origins and his fanciful revolutionary ideas.

In August 1820 the despairing Keats wrote to his beloved Fanny Brawne expressing distress at the parting this would bring:

> I see nothing but thorns for the future—wherever I will be next winter in Italy or nowhere.... Suppose me in Rome—well, I should see you there as in a magic glass going to and from town at all hours.... I wish I was either in your arms full of faith or that a Thunder bolt would strike me.[6]

Keats was concerned about his future and his chances of survival. He wrote to John Taylor, a bookseller, on August 14, 1820. The purpose of this letter was to ask Taylor to make arrangements for his passage on a suitable vessel. He added a postscript to the letter expressing his desires for disposition of his meager estate.

> In case of my death this scrap of Paper may be servic[e]-able in your possession. All of my estate real and personal consists in the hopes of the sale of books publish'd or unpublish'd. Now I wish Brown and you to be the first paid Creditors—the rest is in nubibus—but in case it should shower pay my Taylor the few pounds I owe him. My Chest of Books divide among my friends.[7]

Charles Brown was still in Scotland. Keats hoped to make contact with him; indeed, Keats hoped he would accompany him to Italy. On August 20 he wrote to Brown indicating that he hoped to be *en route* to Italy within a month. This was followed by an undated letter reporting,

> I ought to be off by the end of this week,...but I will wait till I have your answer to this. I am to be introduced before I set out, to a Dr. Clark, a physician settled in Rome, who promises to befriend me in every way.[8]

Brown did not receive these letters. He was already on shipboard heading back to London. In fact, he narrowly missed Keats, as his ship entered the Thames about the same time that Keats was on shipboard heading out. It was Keats's longtime friend Joseph Severn who accompanied the poet to Italy.

On September 17, 1820, Keats and Severn embarked on the *Maria Crowther* bound for Naples. Keats took with him a lock of Fanny Brawne's hair in a locket. Two other passengers occupied the cabin with the men. A Miss Cotterell, also a victim of tuberculosis headed for Italy for her health, and a Mrs. Pidgeon accompanying her. The voyage to Italy was a difficult one. The *Maria Crowther* was forced to turn back by stormy weather and spent many days in the Thames estuary. Once at sea, it encountered another storm in the Bay of Biscay.

The passengers were seasick, especially the two women. When they finally arrived in Naples on October 21, the ship was quarantined in the harbor for ten days because of an outbreak of cholera in England. Early in the voyage while on board the *Maria Crowther*, Keats wrote his last sonnet.

Bright star, would I were stedfast as thou art—
Not in lone splendour hung aloft the night
And watching, with eternal lids apart,
Like nature's patient, sleepless Eremite,
The moving waters at their priest like task
Of pure ablution round earth's human shores,
Or gazing on the new soft-fallen mask
Of snow upon the mountains and the moors —
No — yet still stedfast, still unchangeable,
Pillow'd upon my fair love's ripening breast,
To feel for ever its soft fall and swell,
Awake for ever in a sweet unrest,
Still, still to hear her tender-taken breath,
And so live ever—or else swoon to death.[9]

Death "pillowed on my fair love's ripening breast." A romantic image of death for the poet who knew what awaited him.

After a few days in Naples, Keats and Severn traveled to Rome and met Dr. Clark, who arranged accommodations for them. Keats sickened further, suffering from abdominal complaints that led Clark to be concerned more about those symptoms than about his pulmonary tuberculosis. Perhaps Keats's tuberculosis had spread to his intestinal tract, an event that is rarely seen today but that sometimes occurred late in the course of untreated disease. Severn cared for Keats as he became weaker and obviously close to death. Tuberculosis was generally considered contagious in southern Europe—it was not considered so in Britain and northern Europe—and Severn was faced with the potential cost of burning all of their apartment's furnishings after Keats passed.

Keats was trained in medicine, and his attitude towards his

tuberculosis and impending death reflected that training. His romantic poetry dealt with beauty and love and only rarely death; his letters with reality. Through all, there was a tone of submission to the inevitability of death. Stanza VI of "Ode to a Nightingale," written in May 1819, three months after his portentous blood-spitting, greeted death as "easeful." It may represent the most romantic image of inescapable death written by Keats and was one of a very few such.

Darkling I listen; and, for many a time
I have been half in love with easeful Death,
Call'd him soft names in many a mused rhyme,
To take into the air my quiet breath;
Now more than ever seems it rich to die,
To cease upon the midnight with no pain,
While thou art pouring forth thy soul abroad
In such an ecstasy!
Still wouldst thou sing, and I have ears in vain—
To thy high requiem become a sod.[10]

A letter to Charles Brown written from Naples on November 1, 1820, dealt with his grief at separation from his beloved Fanny Brawne.[11] He clearly anticipated his demise in Italy: "O that I could be buried near where she lives!" This was followed later in the letter by: "Remember me to all. I will endeavour to bear my miseries patiently." There was nothing in this or other letters to suggest that Keats viewed death with any attitude other than resignation.

—

Keats longed for "easeful death." In his medically trained yet romantic mind there could be no outcome to tuberculosis other than death. While he surely was pained by this fatal prognosis, he equally surely accepted it. Resignation and acceptance were the only options for consumptive persons in Keats's era. References to death in his poetry were romantic, to be sure, but they also bespoke the certainty of life's end as the only outcome for the sufferer from tuberculosis.

As the end neared, Keats asked Severn for laudanum (tincture of opium), with which he intended to end his life. Severn refused. On Friday afternoon, February 23, 1821, the twenty-five-year-old Keats died in his friend's arms. An autopsy confirmed the presence of extensive pulmonary and widely disseminated tuberculosis. John Keats was buried in a Protestant cemetery, a letter from Fanny Brawne placed over his heart.

CHAPTER 3

THE CONSUMPTIVE BRONTËS

1814–1855

—Deliverance—

We must all die one day and the illness which is removing me is not painful.

—*Charlotte Brontë,* Jane Eyre

AMONG THE most remarkable of the great Victorian novelists were Anne, Emily, and Charlotte Brontë. Their classic works say much about the lives of their contemporaries, as least as they knew them. A considerable portion of their output came from ideas developed at a time when they were sequestered at their father's parsonage and the Yorkshire village of Haworth. Despite this isolation, they were educated and well read. They worked as governesses. They aspired to be teachers. But they were separated from the lives of other residents of Haworth, a town then experiencing the changes wrought by the industrial revolution. Later, when her literary reputation was established, Charlotte emerged from the cocoon to which the three sisters had been consigned and became established as a popular and respected author. Tuberculosis took the lives of her two sisters before they could emerge into the literary world that accorded their novels posthumous recognition; it spared Charlotte for much of the ensuing decade.

Tuberculosis stalked the members of the Brontë family. As it claimed one life after another, the Brontës never doubted its role as "Captain of all these Men of Death."[1] Emily and Charlotte wrote of tuberculosis in their novels, *Wuthering Heights* and *Jane Eyre.* Charlotte and Anne chronicled the ravages of tuberculosis in the family in the many letters they wrote. These writings, both the novels and the letters, reveal the resignation with which the Brontë sisters viewed the inexorable course of tuberculosis to death. It was clear to them that there was no escape from the disease. With this resignation came despair but also the belief that inescapable death would bring welcome relief and deliverance from suffering.

—

In 1820 the Reverend Patrick Brontë brought his family to Haworth, Yorkshire, where he had accepted a call to become the Evangelical Methodist pastor. There they lived in the parsonage, which stands today as a museum devoted to this remarkable literary family. Patrick Brontë had a chronic cough, which was attributed to bronchitis. One wonders if he had tuberculosis and was the source of the infections in the rest of his family; in fact, this scenario seems probable. It spared him, however, and he lived to the age of eighty-four. His wife, Maria, was not so fortunate. She died at age thirty-eight, a year and eight months after giving birth to the sixth of their children. The cause of her death is not certain. Septicemia following pregnancy and cancer have been suggested by some scholars, but there is little evidence to support either hypothesis. Elizabeth Gaskell, Charlotte Brontë's friend and, following her death, her biographer, wrote that Maria Branwell Brontë's "illness—an internal cancer—... grew and gathered upon her, not many months after her arrival at Haworth."[2] This brief statement by Gaskell appears to be the source for many subsequent references to cancer in Maria Branwell Brontë. The source of this information was probably discussions with Patrick Brontë at the time Gaskell wrote her biography, some thirty-five years after the event. Maria Branwell Brontë became reclusive and morose following the birth of her youngest daughter, perhaps suffering from post-partum depression, but she did not become seriously ill for more than a year thereafter. In the circumstances of the Brontë family, tuberculosis seems likely to have caused her death. In fact, one nineteenth-century author describes her as "consumptive"—frail and weak—from the time when she arrived at Haworth.[3]

All six of the Brontë children died of tuberculosis. The first to succumb was eleven-year-old Maria, who died in May 1825, followed six weeks later by ten-year-old Elizabeth. There are no surviving accounts of their illnesses by health professionals, although they were seen by local doctors, but their symptoms as known are most compatible with tuberculosis. The other children grew to young adulthood. Two decades after his sisters' demises, in September of 1848, Branwell, the only son, died of the disease, his death perhaps hastened by alcoholism and opium addiction; he was thirty-one years old. The Captain of Death waited no more than three months to strike again. Thirty-year-old Emily fell victim in December of that year, and the following spring death came to Anne at age twenty-nine. Charlotte, the last survivor of the children, lived to be age thirty-eight before she passed on with tuberculosis in 1855.

Charlotte, Anne, and Emily Brontë all achieved enduring fame as authors. Their work is often colored by images of consumption, the wasting form of tuberculosis. They had watched their young sisters die of this disease, and all three sisters may have been suffering from its symptoms as they wrote. Emily was the first of the literary trio to fall victim to the disease. Most critics agree that Emily was the most talented of the three, producing poetry and her classic novel, *Wuthering Heights.* It is a brooding, somber tale of degradation and evil, finally—and just barely—triumphed over by love. Revenge yields to redemption. Death is a recurring theme, and while causes of death are not always clear, the courses of disease are lingering and death is seen as a welcome release from long suffering.

> In course of time, Mr. Earnshaw began to fail. He had been active and healthy, yet his strength left him.... But the hour came, at last, that ended Mr. Earnshaw's troubles on earth. He died quietly in his chair one October evening, seated by the fireside.[4]

The death of Earnshaw's wife, Frances, mother of Hareton, a central character in the novel, is described early in the book, setting the somber tone that characterizes so much of the work. It is specifically attributed to tuberculosis. When first seen, she is described in the romanticized image—"young, and fresh complexioned"—so often attributed to tuberculosis sufferers in the nineteenth century.

> She was rather thin, but young, and fresh complexioned, and her eyes sparkled as bright as diamonds. I did remark, to be sure, that mounting the stairs made her breath very quick; that the least sudden noise set her all in a quiver, and that she coughed troublesomely sometimes: but I knew nothing of what these symptoms portended, and had no impulse to sympathize with her.

Later it is made clear to us that the young woman is, indeed, a victim of tuberculosis. Her death is inevitable. But to the moment of her death, she has a "gay heart"; she does not fear—perhaps even welcomes—the inescapable outcome.

> The doctor says she must go: he says she's been in a consumption these many months. I heard him tell Mr. Hindley: and now she has nothing to keep her, and she'll be dead before winter....
>
> Poor soul! Till within a week of her death that gay heart never failed her.... But one night...in the act of saying she thought she should be able to get up to-morrow, a fit of coughing took her—a very slight one...her faced changed, and she was dead.

When death comes to Mr. Linton, Mrs. Dean, the narrator of much of the story, relates her feelings on death, feelings that must surely have reflected those of Emily Brontë.

> I am seldom otherwise than happy while watching in the chamber of death, should no frenzied or despairing mourner share the duty with me. I see a repose that neither earth nor hell can break, and I feel an assurance of the endless and shadowless hereafter—the Eternity they have entered—

> where life is boundless in its duration, and love in its sympathy, and joy in its fullness.

In these passages, illness is seen as chronic, with protracted suffering, and death as both inevitable and a welcome deliverance from suffering. This view certainly reflects Emily's experiences with tuberculosis as a cause of mortality and perhaps her own anticipated passing. Yet, while ill, the suffering person displays a lustrous, romantic quality of beauty: "...her eyes sparkled as bright as diamonds."

Emily Brontë's descriptions of death in *Wuthering Heights* must be read in the context of her own struggles with tuberculosis. While Emily's death certificate described her illness as of only two months' duration, she was ill for a much longer time, probably measured in years, and undoubtedly knew both her diagnosis and her likely outcome. It is not known just when Emily Brontë began or completed *Wuthering Heights*. The work was published in 1847, but much of it was probably written two, or perhaps three, years earlier, when she probably was experiencing symptoms of tuberculosis. Moreover, she had witnessed the deaths of her two sisters, Maria and Elizabeth, when she was a child of seven, and she had nursed her brother as he fell ill and died earlier in the year of her death. As it was for so many persons in the nineteenth century, tuberculosis was a constant and well-known presence. One could only face it with resignation.

Scholars have generally interpreted *Wuthering Heights* as reflecting much more than its story. Some of the malignant aspects of human nature are reflected in the novel; evil pervades the narrative. There is, perhaps, another way of reading *Wuthering Heights* that has not been suggested by literary critics and that may be pertinent to the Brontë family's struggles with tuberculosis, struggles very familiar to Emily Brontë, and a struggle she herself was probably entering upon as she wrote. *Wuthering Heights* can be read as an allegory for the ravages of tuberculosis. Heathcliffe can be viewed as the pervasive, dread disease striking down one by one the members of the Earnshaw and Linton families.

Many of the details of Emily Brontë's decline are portrayed in the writings of her sister, Charlotte. Charlotte was a prolific writer of letters, and she often wrote of her sister's illness. In late October 1848, she penned a letter about Emily to her close friend, Ellen Nussey:

> Emily's cold and cough are very obstinate. I fear she has pain in the chest and I sometimes catch a shortness in her breathing, when she has moved at all quickly. She looks very, very thin and pale. Her reserved nature occasions me great uneasiness of mind. It is useless to question her—you get no answers. It is still more useless to recommend remedies—they are never adopted.[5]

Charlotte Brontë corresponded frequently with Ellen Nussey. In an undated letter written in 1848 she wrote:

> Emily continues much the same; yesterday I thought her a little better, but to-day she is not so well. I hope still—for I must hope—she is dear to me as life—if I let the faintness of despair reach my heart I shall become worthless. The attack was, I believe, in the first place, inflammation of the lungs; it ought to have been met promptly in time. She is too intractable. I do wish I knew her state and feelings more clearly. The fever is not so high as it was, but the pain in the side, the cough, the emaciation are there still.[6]

This was followed on November 23, 1848, by further news of Emily's illness.

> I told you Emily was ill, in my last letter. She has not rallied yet. She is very ill. I believe, if you were to see her, your impression would be that there is not hope. A more hollow, wasted, pallid aspect, I have not beheld. The deep tight cough continues; the breathing after the least exertion is a rapid pant; and these symptoms are accompanied by pains in the chest and side. Her pulse, the only time she allowed it to be felt, was found to beat 115 per minute... God only knows how all this is to terminate.[7]

On December 18, 1848, Charlotte wrote:

> I should have written to you before, if I had had one word of hope to say; but I had not. [Emily] grows daily weaker. The physician's opinion was expressed too obscurely to be of use. He sent some medicine which she would not take. Moments so dark as these I have never known. I pray for God's support to us all.[8]

With what grief Charlotte watched her sister decline. With what hopelessness. How entrapped by the fatal snare was Emily. Yet while wasting, Emily faced her illness calmly with a spirit that was "stronger than a man, simpler than a child."

In her introduction to an early edition on *Wuthering Heights*, Charlotte describes what was probably the terminal dissemination of tuberculosis, which so often brought an end to the chronic disease:

> But a great change approached. Affliction came in that shape which to anticipate is dread; to look back on grief. In the very heat and burden of the day, the laborers failed over their work. My sister Emily…declined. The details of her illness are deep-branded in my memory, but to dwell on them, either in thought or narrative, is not in my power. Never in all her life had she lingered over any task that lay before her, and she did not linger now. She sank rapidly. She made haste to leave us. Yet, while physically she perished, mentally she grew stronger than we had yet known her. Day by day, when I saw with what a front she met suffering, I looked on her with an anguish of wonder and love. I have seen nothing like it; but, indeed, I have never seen her parallel in anything. Stronger than a man, simpler than a child, her nature stood alone. The awful point was that while full of ruth for others, on herself she had no pity; the spirit was inexorable to the flesh; from the trembling hand, the unnerved limbs, the faded eyes, the same service was exacted as they had rendered in health. To stand by and witness

this, and not dare to remonstrate, was a pain no words can render.

Two cruel months of hope and fear passed painfully by, and the day came at last when the terrors and pains of death were to be undergone by this treasure, which had grown dearer and dearer to our hearts as it wasted before our eyes. Towards the decline of that day, we had nothing of Emily but her mortal remains as consumption left them. She died December 19, 1848.[9]

On December 23, 1848, Charlotte wrote to Ellen Nussey once again with the news that Emily had died.

> Emily suffers no more from pain or weakness now. She will never suffer more in this world. She is gone, after a hard, short conflict. She died on Tuesday, the very day I wrote to you.... The anguish of seeing her suffer is over.... We feel she is at peace.[10]

Charlotte wrote to William Smith Williams, the publisher who had first recognized the Brontë sisters' literary talents and a friend with whom she maintained a long correspondence, telling him of Emily's death.

> Emily is nowhere here now—her wasted remains are taken out of the house; we have laid her cherished head under the church aisle beside my mother's, my two sisters', dead long ago, and my poor, hapless brother's....
>
> Well, the loss is ours, not hers, and some sad comfort I take, as I hear the wind blow and feel the cutting keenness of the frost, in knowing that the elements bring her no more suffering—their severity cannot reach her grave—her fever is quieted, her restlessness soothed, her deep hollow cough is hushed forever; we do not hear it in the night nor listen for it in the morning; we have not the conflict of the strangely strong spirit and the fragile frame before us—

> relentless conflict—once seen, never to be forgotten. A dreary calm reigns round us, in the midst of which we seek resignation.[11]

—

It would not be long before the Captain of Death would claim another Brontë. Anne would soon succumb. In the same letter in which Charlotte told Ellen Nussey of Emily's death, she wrote: "I now look to Anne, and wish she were well and strong; but she is neither." On January 15, 1849, she reported:

> I can scarcely say that Anne is worse, nor can I say she is better. She varies often in the course of a day, yet each day is passed pretty much the same. The morning is usually the best time; the afternoon and evening the most feverish. Her cough is the most troublesome at night, but it is rarely violent.[12]

Anne, herself, wrote to Ellen Nussey on April 15, 1849. She was contemplating a trip to the seaside in hopes that it might improve her health.

> The doctors say that a change of air or removal to a better climate would hardly ever fail of success in consumptive cases, if the remedy be taken in time; but the reason why there are so many disappointments is that it is generally deferred till it is too late. Now I would not commit this error; and, to say the truth, though I suffer much less from pain and fever than I did when you were with us, I am decidedly weaker, and very much thinner. My cough still troubles me a good deal, especially in the night, and, what seems worse than all, I am subject to great shortness of breath on going up stairs or any slight exertion. Under these circumstances, I think there is not time to be lost. I have no horror of death: if I thought it inevitable, I think I could quietly resign myself to the prospect.... But I wish it would please God to spare me not only for Papa's and Charlotte's sakes, but because I

> long to do some good in the world before I leave it.... But God's will be done.[13]

Anne did go to the seaside at Scarborough. And on June 4, 1849, Charlotte wrote W. S. Williams, "[Anne] died without a severe struggle, resigned, trusting in God—thankful for release from a suffering life."[14] As Charlotte grieved over this second consumptive death within six months, how must she have felt about the inevitability of tuberculosis, about the Captain of Death that stalked the Brontë family, and about her own future.

Unlike her two sisters, Anne did not specifically include death from tuberculosis in her novels. However, in *The Tenant of Wildfell Hall*, she did write of death, portraying it as a welcome deliverance. "[Death] came quietly upon her, and she was glad to reach her journey's end."[15]

—

Charlotte Brontë, the longest-lived of the Brontë siblings, would die of tuberculosis at age thirty-eight. Her most successful novel was *Jane Eyre*. Much of it reflects Charlotte Brontë's own life as a governess and as a young woman in a frustrated love situation. She wrote of death and tuberculosis in *Jane Eyre*. The early portion of the novel depicts Jane at Lowood School, a boarding school that is generally thought to be based on Cowan Bridge School and the experience of the Brontë sisters at that school. In fact, most scholars believe that Jane Eyre's experiences at Lowood are loosely autobiographical of Charlotte Brontë at Cowan Bridge. In the novel, Jane's best friend, Helen Burns, who is commonly thought to represent Charlotte's sister, Maria, dies of tuberculosis. Jane, who represents Charlotte, visits her in the school infirmary the day before her demise.

> "Helen!" I whispered softly; "are you awake?"
>
> She stirred herself, put back the curtain, and I saw her face, pale, wasted, but quite composed: she looked so little changed that my fear was instantly dissipated....
>
> "I came to see you, Helen: I heard you were very ill, and I could not sleep till I had spoken to you."

> "You came to bid me good-bye, then: you are just in time probably....
>
> "I am very happy, Jane; and when you hear that I am dead, you must be sure and not grieve: there is nothing to grieve about. We all must die one day, and the illness which is removing me is not painful; it is gentle and gradual: my mind is at rest. I leave no one to regret me much.... By dying young, I shall escape great sufferings....
>
> "How comfortable I am! That last fit of coughing has tired me a little; I feel as if I could sleep...."[16]

On June 29, 1854, Charlotte Brontë married the Reverend Arthur Nicholls. Nicholls was the associate pastor in Patrick Brontë's Haworth church and a frequent visitor at the Brontë household. In January 1855, Charlotte became ill, possibly beset by morning sickness of pregnancy, more certainly by fever and cough that surely marked the onset of another episode in her recurrent tuberculosis. Some have suggested that the illness that would cause her death was *hyperemesis gravidarum*, the pernicious, intractable vomiting of pregnancy. However, there is substantial doubt that she was pregnant, and cough was a prominent symptom of her terminal illness. Although her death certificate stated that her "consumption" was of two months' duration, she probably had had intermittent bouts of pulmonary tuberculosis for much of her adult life.

On February 15, 1855, Charlotte penciled a note from her sickbed to Laetitia Wheelwright, a school friend. "At present I am confined to my bed with illness, and have been so for three weeks.... I cannot write more now; for I am much reduced and very weak."[17] Writing again to Ellen Nussey—the final letter from her prolific hand, written lying in her bed, too ill to sit up—she described herself as an emaciated skeleton, and wrote, "I cannot talk—even to my dear, patient, constant Arthur, I can say but a few words at once."[18] Charlotte Brontë died on March 31, 1855, the last of the Brontë family to succumb to tuberculosis.

—

The Brontë family experience with tuberculosis was unusual in that it took so many of them, but the disease was everywhere present in the Europe in which they lived. The writings of the Brontë sisters reflected the attitudes towards and perceptions of tuberculosis of middle-class, educated Britons and Europeans of their time as they faced this overwhelming disease. The Brontë sisters may have been exceptional in anticipating the onset of tuberculosis as inevitable, but their contemporaries generally viewed the Captain of Death, once present, with the same hopelessness as did the three novelist sisters.

Resignation, romanticization, expected release in death, and serene acceptance—despair and ultimately deliverance—these were the inevitable responses of Emily, Anne, and Charlotte Brontë and most victims of tuberculosis in the nineteenth century. What else could one feel in the face of an extraordinarily prevalent, often consumptive disease for which neither cause nor cure were known. Above all and constantly pervasive, despair in the face of a hopeless prognosis for a chronic and debilitating, relentlessly progressive, consuming, fatal disease. Only inevitable death brought deliverance.

CHAPTER 4

NATURALIST

HENRY DAVID THOREAU, 1817–1862

—*Acceptance*—

There is one consolation in being sick, and that is the possibility that you may recover to a better state than you were ever in before.

—*Henry David Thoreau,*
Letter to Harrison G. O. Blake, June 27, 1855

HENRY DAVID THOREAU was a free-thinker, a transcendentalist, a naturalist, a liberal abolitionist. He was a writer of essays about nature and a lecturer who spoke of his travels in the natural world. In these venues he was popular and sought after in his time. An outdoorsman, he gladly suffered physical deprivation and discomfort to be close to nature. He was also a victim of tuberculosis, afflicted with its symptoms intermittently during his active life and ultimately succumbing to it.

David Henry Thoreau—he changed his name to Henry David Thoreau as an adult—was born in Concord, Massachusetts, on July 12, 1817. His father, John Thoreau, and his mother, Cynthia Dunbar Thoreau, had four children, David Henry being the third. Cynthia Thoreau was a liberal thinker and active in her community in Concord. She dominated the Thoreau household. John Thoreau was generally amiable but passive, yielding to his wife in family matters. He was forced to sell the family farm to meet his debts about a year after his son's birth, and he then opened a general store, an enterprise at which he was notably unsuccessful. The family fortunes changed, however, when Charles Thoreau, John's brother, staked a claim to a graphite mine in New Hampshire and brought his brother into the business of producing pencil lead. Their graphite was of a superior quality and the business prospered. The Thoreau family life was generally happy as the pencil business brought financial stability.

Thoreau attended the Concord Academy, graduating in 1833, and then entered Harvard College. He passed the entrance exams with some difficulty. The curriculum at Harvard was based in the classics and included Greek and Latin. Thoreau enjoyed the study of languages, and he studied Italian, French, Spanish, and German. He was an above-average student; at the end of his second term he ranked sixteenth out of a class of about fifty.

In the spring of 1836 Thoreau became ill with tuberculosis, and on May 21 of that year he left Harvard to return to Concord. The Thoreau family had been and would continue to be stalked by tuberculosis, the white plague. It had claimed Thoreau's paternal grandfather. It would take the life of his older sister, Helen, at age thirty-six in 1849. In 1857 it would kill his father. Tuberculosis also afflicted his brother, John, who would die not of tuberculosis but of tetanus incurred following a wound. Thoreau recovered his health while sojourning in Concord. "My health is so much improved that I shall return to [Harvard] next term if they will receive me," he wrote in a letter to a friend.[1] He did return to Harvard in the fall of 1836. He completed his final year, and received his diploma at the annual commencement exercises on August 31, 1837.

During the next few years Thoreau sought positions as a school teacher or tutor, but failed to establish himself in that profession. He obtained a position teaching at the Center School in Concord following his graduation from Harvard, but resigned shortly thereafter when he was confronted by the school committee over his refusal to employ corporal punishment—whipping—to discipline his young students. He worked in the family pencil business, and he introduced innovations into the compounding of graphite with clay to make pencil leads superior to those of competitors. Thoreau achieved this advance by researching the methods used in Germany at the Harvard library.

In September 1835 Ralph Waldo Emerson moved to Concord.

He befriended Thoreau and lent him books from his large library. Emerson became the leader of the transcendentalist movement in America. Originating in the seventeenth-century writings of John Locke, transcendentalism espoused the view that "would we but obey that light within us we could attain a fulfillment, a happiness, and a success such as man has never known."[2]

At age twenty-two, Thoreau fell in love with Ellen Sewall during a visit of her family to the Thoreaus in the summer of 1839. He wrote poetry to her and proposed marriage. So also did his brother, John, seek the young woman's hand. She spurned them both, however. Two years later he was again smitten by the arrow of Cupid; this time Mary Russell, who was serving as a governess in the Emerson household, captured his attention. More poetry followed, but once again his suit was unsuccessful. Thereafter Thoreau remained single without further amorous relationships.

Retreats to nature were a frequent and sometimes constant part of Thoreau's life. With one or more friends, he trekked and camped throughout New England. Sometimes he traveled by foot, sometimes in small boats or canoes on rivers. Cape Cod, the Berkshire Mountains of Massachusetts, the White Mountains of New Hampshire, and the Moosehead and Allagash Lake wilderness areas of Maine all were destinations. He climbed and camped on Mount Greylock, Mount Katahdin, and Mount Washington. Not infrequently he spent cold and stormy nights in primitive shelters. Most famously, he retreated to Walden Pond, not far from Concord, in the spring of 1845. There he built a small, primitive cabin on land owned by Emerson. It was his home for the ensuing two years. These outdoor excursions testify to Thoreau's vigorous good health at that time in his life. At Walden he first took up surveying; later he would find employment as a surveyor, contributing thus to his income.

Increasingly, Thoreau turned his efforts to writing. He began keeping a journal in October 1837, filling it with observations on the world that surrounded him. Many of his early essays on nature and on observations made during his travels were published in *The Dial*, a transcendentalist journal edited by Emerson. He published books, the most famous of which, *Walden*, was begun while he was at

Walden Pond. After many revisions, it was finally published in 1854. Success of this book led to invitations to give lectures, although Thoreau was disappointed that the number of these lectures fell short of his views of his stature as a lecturer.

Thoreau was in ill health for about two years in 1855 through 1857. On June 27, 1855 he wrote to Harrison Blake, a close friend since their student years together at Harvard, describing his illness.

> I have been sick and good for nothing but to lie on my back and wait for something to turn up, for two or three months. This has compelled me to postpone several things.... I should feel a little less ashamed if I could give any name to my disorder, but I cannot, and our doctor cannot help me to it, and I will not take the name of any disease in vain. However, there is one consolation in being sick, and that is the possibility that you may recover to a better state than you were ever in before. I expected in the winter to be deep in the woods of Maine in my canoe long before this, but I am so far from that that I can only take a languid walk in Concord streets.[3]

The nature of Thoreau's illness may have eluded the doctor who "could not help [him] to it." In fact, some modern biographers have been puzzled by this illness and considered his symptoms psychoneurotic. It is difficult, however, for a modern medical reader cognizant of the natural history of tuberculosis not to conclude that Thoreau's tuberculosis had reactivated at this time.

Thoreau's health returned. In the spring of 1858 he was well enough to resume activities as a surveyor. The summer of 1858 found him roaming New England forests again. In June he climbed Mount Monadnock; in July, Mount Washington. His good health continued, and the summer of 1860 was once again passed on mountain trails. He was active as a lecturer at this time.

Tuberculosis returned to Thoreau late in 1860. He spent most of the ensuing winter confined to the house, and lapses appeared in his daily journaling. In December he was given a diagnosis of "bronchitis," almost certainly a manifestation of his reactivated tuberculosis. He improved somewhat in the spring of 1861 and was able to take brief walks in Concord.

Thoreau's doctors advised him to travel to a warm climate, a common prescription of the time for those who suffered from tuberculosis. The Caribbean and the Mediterranean Riviera were popular destinations and were recommended to him, but they seemed beyond his fiscal means. He decided to go to Minnesota, a state alleged to have beneficially dry air. His usual travel companions were not available, and he enlisted Horace Mann, Jr. (son of the educator) to accompany him. The rail trip was arduous for Thoreau. He spent the summer in Minneapolis, living in the boarding house of widow Elizabeth Hamilton on the south shore of Lake Calhoun.[4] The building no longer stands; Andreas Ueland bought the property in 1884 and replaced it with a large home for his growing family of four children in 1885. Thoreau explored the Linden Hills district of Minneapolis, including nearby Lake Harriet. He improved somewhat. He was intrigued to see plant and small animal species not familiar to him in New England. He made a side trip to an Indian settlement in Northern Minnesota. In July Thoreau and Mann returned to Concord, traveling by steamer on the Great Lakes for much of the homeward journey.

As cold and snow returned to Concord, Thoreau's health ebbed. Winter found him sick in bed. It soon became apparent to all that he would not long survive. Thoreau's spirits did not flag, however, but he was too weak to continue his usual activities. On February 11, he wrote to the editors of *The Atlantic Monthly* concerning the publication of some of his work.

> Only extreme illness has prevented my answering your note earlier. I have no objection to having the papers you refer to printed in your monthly—if my feeble health will permit me to prepare them for the printer.[5]

Soon thereafter he was dictating his correspondence to his sister, Sophia, as he was too ill to write himself.

Henry David Thoreau died on the evening of May 6, 1862.

One must ask what Thoreau thought of his chronic, relapsing, and relentlessly advancing tuberculosis. Certainly it did not dim his enthusiasm for life or his desire to live his life in the fullest of measures he could envision. He did not write of his disease in his daily journal, confining the entries on those pages to descriptions of the natural world surrounding him. Yet he accepted his illness, resigned to it. Thoreau appears to have put his own mortality out of his mind. However, the sudden death of his brother in January 1842 from tetanus following a wound had a profound impact on him. He found himself grieving without the comfort afforded to many by religion, which his transcendentalist views had swept away. Two and one-half years earlier, in September 1839, the two brothers had taken a boat trip on the Concord and Merrimack Rivers. Both were suffering from tuberculosis at the time, but they were well enough to enjoy the rigors of rowing, camping, and side trips up mountain slopes. Thoreau conceived of a book to honor his brother. The work that emerged is much more than a journal or travelogue. Thoreau reflects on nature and on the human condition. Portions of the first draft were written in 1842. A second draft contained many revisions. Thoreau could not find a publisher willing to put it into print. Finally, after much further revision, *A Week on the Concord and Merrimack Rivers* was completed at Walden in 1845. Thoreau published it at his own expense; it did not sell well.

While not dealing specifically with tuberculosis, Thoreau's attitude towards death is revealed in this work, especially in the first draft, which contains portions not included in later versions.

> Truly the gods are kind. Though natural laws are more immutable than any despots yet to our daily life they rarely seem rigid, but permit us to relax with license in summer weather. We are not often nor harshly reminded of the things we may not do. I am often astonished to see how long and often after what manifold infringements of the natural laws some men maintain life. She certainly does not deny them quarter, they do not die without priest— And what does she care, in any case they are sure not to depart out

> of her demesnes.— It would seem as if consistency were the secret of health. How many a pure man—striving to live a pure life pines and dies after a life of sickness, and his friends wonder if nature is not pitiless.[6]

Perhaps Thoreau's attitude towards his disease is best epitomized by paragraphs from a letter to his friend Harrison Blake dated December 6, 1856. He was ill at that time, although it is not clear that he knew his illness was once again tuberculosis.

> For my part I am trying to wake up,—to wring slumber out of my pores;— For, generally, I take events as unconcernedly as a fence post,—absorb wet & cold like it, and am pleasantly tickled with lichens slowly spreading over me. Could I not be content then to be a cedar post, which lasts 25 years? Would I not rather be that than the farmer that set it? or he that preaches to that farmer?—& go to the heaven of posts at last? I think I should like that as well as any would like it. But I should not care if I sprouted into a living tree, put forth leaves & flowers, & have fruit.
>
> I am grateful for what I am & have. My thanksgiving is perpetual. It is surprising how contented one can be with nothing definite.[7]

Thoreau did not see justice in the fate he surely knew would be his. He seems to ask, "Why me?" Yet he was ready to accept what awaited him—to accept it resignedly, as a fence post must accept its fate, wet, cold, covered in lichens, or sprouting new branches of life.

CHAPTER 5

VOICE OF THE SOUTH

SIDNEY CLOPTON LANIER, 1842–1881

—Struggle—

My soul shall float, friend Sun,
The day being done.

—Sidney Clopton Lanier, Sunrise

SIDNEY CLOPTON Lanier is remembered as one of America's greatest romantic poets. He was born into the gracious antebellum world of the early nineteenth-century, agricultural, American South. He suffered through the ruinous Civil War, as did his homeland region and his fellow Confederate southerners. He struggled to create a life in the post-war period. His seesaw, but relentless and increasingly desperate, battle with tuberculosis dominated his short life. Perhaps his consuming illness can be viewed as a metaphor for the troubled post-Civil War, reconstruction times of his native Georgia and the other Confederate states.

Lanier was born on February 3, 1842 in Macon, Georgia, the first of three children of Robert Sampson Lanier and Mary Jane Anderson Lanier. His father was a lawyer; his mother a talented musician and accomplished pianist. The genealogy of the Lanier family is rooted in French Huguenots; Jerome Lanier fled France to become attached to the court of English Queen Elizabeth. In 1716 Thomas Lanier immigrated to America with a land grant in what is now Richmond, Virginia. Subsequent generations of Laniers settled in many parts of the American South.

At an early age, Lanier's musical talents emerged. Taught largely by his mother, he first essayed the flute at age six and soon could play not only the flute, which would remain his principal instrument throughout his life, but also the guitar, piano, and violin. His schooling was irregular, largely accomplished by tutoring at home, but included a year at the Bibb County Academy. He was admitted to the sophomore year of nearby Oglethorpe College, a Presbyterian college, in January 1857, shortly before his fifteenth birthday. The following year he left college because of ill health, returning to Macon to work as a postal clerk. The nature of this illness as described by his biographers is not clear, but one must suspect that it might have been his initial encounter with the tuberculosis that plagued him throughout his life. He returned to Oglethorpe College in the autumn of 1859 and graduated at the top of his class. His literary talents began to blossom at this time—he started work on a novel—and he continued to shine as a musician. He wrote to his father about his musical talent.

> I am more than all perplexed by this fact, that the prime inclination, that is, natural bent (which I have checked, though) of my nature is to music; and for that I have the greatest talent; indeed, not boasting, for God gave it me, I have an extraordinary musical talent, and feel it is within me plainly that I could rise as high as any composer. But I cannot bring myself to believe that I was intended for a musician, because it seems so small a business in comparison with other things which, it seems to me, I might do.[1]

The "other things which…I might do" comprised, of course, writing poetry.

Lanier was offered a job as a tutor at Oglethorpe College, and he planned to go to Heidelberg, Germany for further study. However, the eruption of the Civil War in 1861 altered his plans, as it did those of so many of America's youth. Together with his brother, Clifford, he enlisted in the Macon Volunteers in July 1861. The two brothers were sent to Richmond—they would serve side by side throughout most of the war—and saw action in several of the battles that occurred in that area. Army camps of that time were frequently plagued with illness, and in Lanier's case it was not so much the ever-present fever and dysentery but his progressing tuberculosis that made him ill. While home on furlough in the spring of 1863 he met Mary Day, who would later become his wife.

In August of 1864 the two brothers were assigned as signal officers on British ships running the blockade. In November his ship was captured. The British crew was released, but Lanier was held and sent to Point Lookout, Maryland, as a prisoner of the Union forces. He hid his flute in his sleeve, and it accompanied him to his jail. At Point Lookout his tuberculosis worsened. In late February of 1865 he was released and made his way back to Macon, sick, sometimes delirious. That summer he accepted a position as a tutor at a nearby plantation, but by October he found himself too ill to continue. "No bone in me but aches, no nerve but tingles when I cough," he wrote to a friend.

Slowly, while resting at home, his health improved. In the summer of 1867 he became engaged to Mary Day; they were married on December 19, 1867. Four weeks later he frightened his bride by coughing up blood in a major episode of hemoptysis. He studied law, passed the bar exam, and in 1869 joined his father's law practice. Throughout this period, he gave flute concerts and wrote, although no completed works were published at this time.

Travel to favorable locations and climates was a frequent prescription for tuberculous patients. In 1870 he set out for Minnesota, following the earlier footsteps of Thoreau to what was said to be a favorable region for consumptives. However, he found himself too ill to continue the journey and returned home. He tried the sea air at Brunswick, Georgia, and a spa at Alleghany Springs, Virginia, but neither proved sufficiently salubrious. Leaving his wife and children behind, he went to San Antonio, Texas, in December 1872. From there he wrote to his wife a letter that looks at death perhaps in despair but also romantically.

> Were it not for some circumstances which made such a proposition seem absurd in the highest degree, I would think that I am shortly to die, and that my spirit has been

> singing its swan-song before dissolution. All day my soul hath been cutting swiftly into the great space of the subtle, unspeakable deep, driven by wind after wind of heavenly melody. The very spirit and essence of all wind-songs, bird-songs, passion-songs, folk-songs, country-songs, sex-songs, soul-songs, and body-songs hath blown upon me in quick gusts like the breath of passion, and sailed me into a sea of vast dreams, whereof each wave is at once a vision and a melody.

The end of 1873 found Lanier in New York and then in Baltimore, Maryland. He was determined to pursue a career in music and poetry. He wrote of his struggle to his father

> My dear father, think how for twenty years, through poverty, through pain, through weariness, through sickness, through the uncongenial atmosphere of a farcical college and of a bare army and then of an exacting business life, through all the discouragement of being wholly unacquainted with literary people and literary ways—I say, think how, in spite of all these depressing circumstances, and of a thousand more which I could enumerate, these two figures of music and poetry have steadily kept in my heart so that I could not banish them.

Despite continued illness and frequent interruptions, Lanier succeeded in pursuing his two dreams. He secured an appointment as the principal flutist at the Peabody Institute Orchestra in Baltimore at a salary of $120 per year. Publishers began to accept his poetry. He finished several books, including some for young people. In 1878 he was made a Lecturer in English Literature at Johns Hopkins University, for which he received an annual salary of $1,000. He and his family were settled in Baltimore in reasonably comfortable circumstances.

In May 1881 Lanier received a $1,500 commission to write about North Carolina and Virginia resorts. He left Baltimore to undertake this task. His tuberculosis followed him, increasingly rendering him ill. He worked on the project and finished some of his most remarkable poems. But the end was at hand. He died in Lynn, North Carolina, on September 7, 1881. He was thirty-nine years old.

—

Although Lanier's letters referred, sometimes obliquely, to his tuberculosis, illness and death were not prominent in his romantic, often lyrical poetry. Most of his poems were couched as hymns of nature. Yet they were written by a man struggling with a disease that, in his time, had about a fifty percent mortality rate. Lanier surely knew this and was aware of the progression of his tuberculosis. He must have expected that he would succumb to the "Captain of all These Men of Death."

Resurrection clearly evokes the image of one wandering through a graveyard. It dates from 1868 when Lanier was resting from a flare up of his tuberculosis and studying law with his father. One is led to envision a resurrected soul free of all of the troubles of life. And yet, the image of a pained and bruised life leading to death is inescapable.

Fair now the brows old Pain had erewhile wrinkled,
And peace and strength about the calm mouth dwell.
Clean of the ashes that Repentance sprinkled,
The meek head poises like a flower-bell.

All the old scars of wanton wars are vanished;
And what blue bruises grappling Sense had left
And sad remains of redder stains are banished,
And the dim blotch of heart-committed theft.[2]

The short, fragmentary, four-line verse, *Struggle*, was probably written in 1978 when he was in Baltimore.

My soul is like the oar that momentarily
Dies in a desperate stress beneath the wave,
Then glitters out again and sweeps the sea;
Each second I'm new-born from some new grave.

Surely these lines reflect Lanier's struggle with tuberculosis—sometimes very ill, sometimes seemingly well.

Lanier's last major poem, written in Baltimore in 1880 as he faced debilitating illness, his last few months of life ebbing away, was *Sunrise*, part of a set of works entitled *Hymns of the Marshes*. They were inspired by the Marshes of Glynn, the wetland that separates the barrier "Golden Isles" from the coast of Georgia near Brunswick. Lanier had visited the area in his attempts to find a climate favorable to healing of his tuberculosis. *Sunrise*, although placed first in the set, was the last written and the last major poem to come from Lanier's pen. Parks argues that, "the marsh had become a symbol in his mind of the condition from which man had developed.... A man was free to make his own choices; he was not a biological pawn in a pre-determined game."[3] His wife called it "the culminating poem, the highest vision."[4]

Sunrise can be read as an allegory. As daylight spreads across the marsh, illuminating one chapter after another of the living tidal wetland, so the span of a life brings one image after another to a person growing from childhood to the last years of life. Some images are bright, some somber.

Reverend Marsh, low-couched along the sea,
Old chemist, rapt in alchemy,
Distilling silence,—lo,
That which our father-age had died to know—
The menstruum that dissolves all matter—thou
Hast found it; for this silence, filling now
The globéd charity of receiving space,
This solves us all: man, matter, doubt, disgrace,
Death, love, sin, sanity,
Must in yon silence, clear solution lie.

The poem closes with what were probably the last lines Lanier penned, his valedictory.

And as ever my heart through the night shall with knowledge
abide thee,
And ever by day shall my spirit, as one that hath tried thee,
Labor, at leisure, in art,—till yonder beside thee
My soul shall float, friend Sun,
The day being done.

CHAPTER 6

DEMI-MONDE

ALEXANDRE DUMAS *FILS*, 1824–1895

—*Resignation*—

> *You will have a sorry mistress; a woman who is nervous, ill, sad, or gay with a gaiety that is sadder than grief, a woman who spits blood.*
>
> —*Alexandre Dumas* fils,
> The Lady of the Camellias

ALTHOUGH EUROPEAN tuberculosis death rates were falling throughout the nineteenth century, they remained extraordinarily high by modern standards. This dread disease was never far from the minds and lives of those who wrote about their times. Alexandre Dumas *fils* produced fiction reflecting the life he led at this time. Giuseppe Verdi converted his work into a popular opera. Indeed, this opera, *La Traviata*, epitomizes a perception of tuberculosis that arose early in the nineteenth century and became prevalent in its later years.

Alexandre Dumas *fils* was a much celebrated, popular author and playwright. His father, Alexandre Dumas *père*, was a noted novelist—*The Three Musketeers* is much remembered among his works—who lived a libertine life style. In 1823, while working as a clerk, the father developed a liaison with Marie Catherine Lebay, a seamstress. Their son was born on July 27, 1824. Not until April 21, 1831, when the boy was six years old, did Dumas *père* publically accept and acknowledge the paternity of his son. Schoolmates taunted the young Dumas because of his illegitimacy; he did not finish secondary school.

At age seventeen, Dumas went to live with his father. The society in which the elder Dumas moved interacted with what Dumas *fils* would later call the *demi-monde*, distinguishing it from high society (*haute monde*) of the time. Courtesans kept by wealthy patrons were a major feature of this stratum of society. These women were attractive, talented, and much courted by wealthy men. They were not prostitutes—they did not expect direct payment for their services—but they lived off the largess of their patrons. One did not keep such a woman without paying all of the costs of her usually extravagant life style.

In September 1844, the twenty-year-old Dumas met Marie Duplessis. They were soon lovers. Marie Duplessis was a remarkable woman. Born Alphonsine Plessis on January 15, 1824, she was the daughter of Marin Plessis, a peddler, and Marie Deshayes Plessis. Her mother died when she was six years old, and she spent the next seven or eight years living with relatives and working in laundries. In 1839, her father took her to Paris, leaving the fifteen-year-old girl with relatives of her mother. They found laundry work for her. That summer Alphonsine met the first of her many lovers, and entered on the life of a courtesan.

Taking the name of Marie Duplessis, the young woman rapidly acquired the skills and manners that made her famous among the courtesans of her world. She was strikingly beautiful and dressed elegantly. She was gracious and charming to all. She was devoted to the theater, attending performances nightly. She learned to play the piano. She danced gracefully. She also spent extravagantly, furnishing a series of apartments provided by her lovers with taste and without sparing costs. She gambled recklessly. She also became ill with tuberculosis. Although she visited spas and felt better after doing so, she was never free of the disease.

Marie Duplessis had a series of lovers and patrons from among the wealthy men of Paris. Alexandre Dumas *fils*, whom she called Adet and who signed his love letters to her AD, entered her orbit in September 1844. Their relationship was marked by genuine love; it was not simply the casual, money-driven liaison of most of her relationships with men. After about a year, Dumas realized that he could no longer afford to maintain his relationship with Marie. On August 30, 1845, he wrote to her breaking off their relationship.

> My dear Marie. I am neither rich enough to love you as I would like nor poor enough to be loved as you would like. So let us both forget—you a name which must mean hardly anything to you—me a happiness which has become impossible to bear. There is no point in telling you how sad I am—for you already know how much I love you. So farewell—you have too great a heart not to understand the reason for my letter and too good a nature not to forgive me for it. A thousand memories. AD[1]

Marie resumed her life as a courtesan. She met and charmed Franz Liszt, who offered to take her with him to Constantinople. In 1846 she married Count Eduard de Perrégaux in London, but never lived with him. Ill with an exacerbation of her tuberculosis, she returned to Paris in September. Her health failed rapidly, and she began selling her possessions to meet her expenses, including doctors' bills. She died on February 3, 1847. She was twenty-three years old. Her personal possessions and household goods were sold at an auction held in her apartment.

—

If one is to believe the author's statements, Dumas's novel, *La Dame aux camélias* (translated into English and retitled *Camille*) was written in three or four weeks at about the time of the first anniversary of Duplessis's death and two and one-half years after the two lovers had separated.[2] It was immediately successful, and was turned into an equally successful play, *La Dame aux camélias*, four years later. Giuseppe Verdi and his librettist, Francesco Maria Piave, soon adapted it for their ever-popular opera, *La Traviata*, which was first performed in March 1853. Within five years this romantic tale had achieved enormous popularity as a book, on the stage as a play, and as one of Verdi's most memorable operas. Much of the story of Marguerite and Armand (in the novel) or Violetta and Alfredo (in the opera) reprises the story of Dumas and Duplessis.

The novel opens with the auction from her apartment of the impoverished Marguerite's possessions after her death from tuberculosis, an account that parallels the facts of Marie Duplessis's demise. The grief-stricken Armand Duval then recounts the tale of his love to a narrator. In brief, Armand fell in love with Marguerite instantly on first seeing her and soon became her lover. She was a courtesan—a "kept woman"—and depended on the largess of her several patrons to maintain her luxurious life style and her gambling addiction. Armand borrowed heavily to support his relationship with her. To this point, the story parallels the actual events of the affair of Dumas and Duplessis. Marguerite discourages Armand's professed love.

> "So you are in love with me.... You will do better never to say it."
>
> "Why?"
>
> "Because only one of two things can come of it."
>
> "What?"
>
> "Either I shall not accept; then you will have a grudge against me; or I shall accept; then you will have a sorry mistress; a woman who is nervous, ill, sad, or gay with a gaiety that is sadder than grief, a woman who spits blood and spends a hundred thousand francs a year."[3]

Armand persists in his love, but ultimately he writes to Marguerite breaking off the relationship that he no longer has sufficient funds to support. This letter is remarkably similar to the actual letter that Dumas wrote to Duplessis. Armand signed it with the initials AD, just as was the Dumas letter to Duplessis.

> Goodbye, my dear Marguerite. I am not rich enough to love you as I would nor poor enough to love you as you would. Let us then forget, you a name which must be indifferent enough to you, I a happiness which has become impossible.

The work continues, departing from its autobiographical mode to further develop its plot along lines that do not reflect the now separate lives of Dumas and Duplessis. The two lovers leave Paris for a cottage in a nearby village. There they live simply and are boundlessly happy. Armand's father intervenes, determined to end his son's extravagant spending, including commitment of his son's portion of the family estate to Marguerite, and desiring to protect the family's small-town reputation so that his daughter can make a favorable marriage. Armand will not listen to his father, but the latter man appeals to Marguerite's generosity and love for Armand. She yields to the father's pleas, and she leaves Armand to return to her life as a courtesan. Her health rapidly failing, she succumbs to tuberculosis. Armand, away from Paris at the Duval family home, finally learns from his father of the role he played in inducing Marguerite to return to Paris. His father urges Armand to return to Paris and reclaim Marguerite. He does so, learns of her death, and finds her possessions being sold at auction.

When adapting his story to the stage, Dumas made important changes that both facilitated its production and increased its dramatic impact.[4] Gone is the device of Armand relating his tale to another, who serves as the narrator. Gone are scenes set in the Bois or the Champs-Elysées. They are replaced by action in Marguerite's quarters. Dumas added a dramatic duel challenge between Armand and the patron to whom Marguerite returned after leaving Armand and their country idyll, although the duel takes place between acts. In the play, Armand, now understanding what has transpired between Marguerite and his father, returns in the final act to hold Marguerite in his arms as she dies. In many other aspects, the play is faithful to the novel, especially as Marguerite attempts to discourage Armand's love. She has resigned herself to sickness and ultimate death, and she does not wish to inflict that sorrow on the man she loves.

The prolific composer of operas, Giuseppe Verdi, and his librettist, Francesco Maria Piave, based their opera, *La Traviata,* on Dumas's story. It is set in Paris in 1840, and the opera does not wander far from Dumas's play. Its premiere in Venice on March 6, 1853, was an unfortunate disaster; the story was thought by many to be immoral, and the production suffered from poor performances by the singers. Subsequently the opera was restaged and performed by a better cast. The emotional impact of the new production was enormous. It was then well received and has since become one of the most popular of all operas.

Adapted from Dumas's work, *La Traviata* generally parallels, while condensing, the play and, accordingly, part of the Dumas-Duplessis romance. Act I is set at a party given by Violetta (Duplessis and Marguerite). Generally a joyous scene, it is punctuated by Violetta's tubercular cough. Alfredo (Dumas and Armand) takes the opportunity provided by a shift in the festivities to an adjoining room to profess his great love to Violetta. As in the novel, he had fallen in love with her instantly when he first saw her a year previously. She teases him, and urges him not to love her.

> *Pure friendship I can give,*
> *but I don't know what love is,...*[5]

Soon, however, Violetta responds to Alfredo's overtures and professes her love for him. Act II opens with Scene 1 set in a country house. There the two lovers are happily ensconced, as in the novel. Alfredo's father arrives and persuades Violetta to leave Alfredo for the sake of Alfredo's young sister's marriage prospects. She writes a farewell letter and returns to Paris. Scene 2 is set back at Violetta's Paris house, where a party is in progress. Alfredo arrives and is told by Violetta that she no longer loves him and has returned to the favor of a baron. Alfredo denounces her. Act III finds Violetta on her death bed. Alfredo has received a letter from his father revealing the part he played in inducing Violetta to return to Paris. Alfredo enters and the two sing of their love and their happy times together. Destroyed by her tuberculosis, Violetta dies in Alfredo's arms.

Resignation in the face of inevitable death from tuberculosis is colored by romanticization in the story of Marguerite and Armand. Like a pyrotechnic display, the life of Dumas's heroine, Marguerite, flared with bright beauty as it sped towards inevitable extinction. However luminous her life and love, her tuberculous death was inescapable. The person stricken with this dread disease could only accept the predictable outcome with resignation. This realization pervades Dumas's story in all three of its versions.

The response of victims of tuberculosis to their illness as portrayed by Dumas in his novel was marked by romanticization, by a "gaiety sadder than grief." Marguerite says to Armand, "You will have a sorry mistress: a woman who is nervous, ill, sad, or gay with a gaiety sadder than grief, a woman who spits blood. . . ."[6] Later in the novel, Marguerite speaks to Armand of her life as a courtesan whose ultimate fate is the inescapable destiny of a victim of tuberculosis. "If one is bound to be consumed, it is as well to throw oneself into the flames as to be asphyxiated with charcoal."[7]

While despairing and in pain on the beach near Naples, Italy, Percy Bysshe Shelley wrote his famous couplet:

I could lie down like a tired child,
And weep away the life of care.[8]

The image of an innocent, tired child evokes a feeling of resignation, of acceptance of impending death. Dumas most certainly had read Shelley's poem. Dumas's genre was prose, not poetry. Yet, one must wonder, was Shelley's verse in his mind when Dumas gave to Armand words describing his despair at the loss of Marguerite: "When I reached home I began to cry like a child"?[9] As Dumas closed his novel, he gave to his protagonist-narrator the words, "I would gladly be the echo of noble sorrow wherever I hear its voice."[10]

—

Resignation is a theme that carries forward from Dumas's work to *La Traviata*. Indeed, the entire work is one of repeated images of the consumptive heroine facing inescapable death, resigned to it. Facing unavoidable death, Violetta sings:

It's too late!
I wait and wait but they'll never come!
Oh, how I have changed!
Yet the Doctor tried to give me hope!
Ah, with this disease all hope is dead!
Farewell to the past; to bright dreams;
The roses in my cheeks are faded.

Close to her last breath, Violetta gives Alfredo a miniature portrait of herself and sings:

And if a gentle maiden in the flower of her youth should give
you her heart,
make her your wife, I wish it.
Then give her this portrait and tell her it is a gift from one
among the angels,
who prays for her and for you.

Violetta is certain that all of her sins will be forgiven and that she will reside among angels.

—

Dumas married Nadesjda von Knorring in 1864 and had two daughters. After his wife's death, he married Henriette Régnier de la Brière in June 1895. Dumas died on November 27, 1895, and was buried in the Montmartre cemetery in Paris, his grave located a scant one hundred yards from that of Marie Duplessis.

Dumas's Marguerite faced inescapable death from tuberculosis. Yet the candles of her life burned brightly. She lived gaily, if not always joyously. She did not, however, deny her illness. She faced her expected demise with resignation that allowed her to continue to laugh and at least mount a mask of happiness. When Verdi surrounded his opera heroine with choruses, ballet corps, and lavish stage sets, the drama of the illness and the fate of its victim became even more prominent. The views of tuberculosis of the composer and librettist are reflected in the opera. But then, one must acknowledge, death is common at the close of operas. That tuberculosis leads to death was an expected outcome at the time, both for the disease and for an opera.

Keats and the Brontë sisters knew tuberculosis personally, and their written images of the disease reflected their despair-filled lives. Dumas did not have tuberculosis. The consumptive woman he took to his heart did, and their love and her disease colored his images. He wrote of a beautiful woman who lived a tragic life, accepting her fate, resigned to it.

CHAPTER 7

BOHEMIA

HENRY MÜRGER, 1822–1861

—*Romanticization*—

You meant to say, beautiful as a sunset.
—*Giacomo Puccini,* La Bohème,
Libretto by Giuseppe Giacosa and Luigi Illica,

AUTHOR, DRAMATIST, and chronicler of nineteenth-century life in the Left Bank Bohemian sector of Paris, Henry Mürger was born Louis-Henri Murger on March 27, 1822. His father, Claude-Gabriel Murger, was a tailor; his mother, Hortense-Henriette, a seamstress. When his father secured an additional position as concierge in a Paris apartment building, the increased income permitted better schooling for the boy. Additionally, the young Murger, called Henri, came into contact with the more affluent residents of the building, who encouraged him to read and to develop an interest in the arts. Murger's father expected his adolescent son to take his place on the tailor's bench and learn that trade. The boy rebelled. With the sympathy of his mother and the help of his apartment house resident friends, he obtained positions initially as a law clerk and later as secretary to Count Tolstoy. Tolstoy liked the boy and supported him—with encouragement and often money—during coming years. The clerk position was not demanding and allowed Murger time to pursue his growing interests in literature and the arts.

Three close friends, Eugène Pottier from his school years, Pierre Brison, and Emile Brison, brothers and fellow law clerks, introduced Murger to the Latin Quarter. Originally a neighborhood of international students at La Sorbonne whose only language in common was

Latin, it had become a district frequented by artists, actors, and writers. Murger dabbled at drawing and painting, for which he had little talent, and began writing poetry. He gained scant recognition as a poet. Later he wrote prose essays and short stories with greater success. He changed his name to the more aristocratic Henry Mürger in February 1845 with the important publication of one of his earliest stories. Following the death of his mother and the loss of her championship at home, Mürger's father became increasingly disaffected by the young man's Bohemian ways. He expelled him from the home, never again to be reconciled with him.

At age eighteen, Mürger fell in love and took the first of several women to his bed chamber. She was Marie Vimal, a pretty, blue-eyed bookkeeper. Age twenty-five, she was seven years older than Henri. She had been recently and unhappily married to a middle-aged accountant named Fontblanc, from whom she was now estranged. Marie took up residence with Henri and taught him English. She would move in and out of his life, changing partners from time to time, but she was never far removed from his heart, although he also would find other women to share his bed. Marie was, in large part, the model for Mimi, the heroine of his *Scènes de la vie de bohème*, the version upon which Puccini's opera, *La Bohème*, is based.

Constantly in debt and moving from garret to garret, Mürger increasingly turned from writing poetry to prose. Many of his days were spent in cafés frequented by his fellow Bohemians, particularly the Café Momus. A cadre of young women called *grisettes* followed these aspiring artists, often shifting partners among them, sometimes serving as models for those who were painters. Perhaps the modern slang term "groupie" as applied to fans of modern rock entertainers might well be applied to these women. The men they idolized were not as successful as modern rock stars, however, and the women's relationships with the men were more intimate than those achieved by most "groupies."

Mürger shared a garret with J. Champfleury and his paramour, Marie Roux, who would serve as the model for Musette in his play, *Vie de la bohème*; his book, *Scènes de la bohème*; and Musetta in the opera, *La Bohème*. Marie Roux introduced Mürger to Lucille Louvet, who soon became his lover. He called her Mimi, and she also would serve as a model for his heroine, Mimi. Lucille/Mimi had tuberculosis and would soon die in a charity ward of the Hôpital St. Louis, not in the arms of her lover as depicted in Mürger's play and in the opera. Mürger soon thereafter took up with another *grisette* named Juliette; she also died of tuberculosis.

In 1845 the publisher of *Corsaire*, a leading periodical devoted to literature, accepted a story by Mürger entitled "Un Envoyé de la providence." This piece would be the first of a series published by *Corsaire* in which Mürger described the life of the Paris Bohemians. His characters were drawn from his acquaintances, often with names changed only slightly; he himself became Rodolphe, Rodolfo in the opera. The settings were those in which Mürger spent his days and nights—the Latin Quarter, his garret, and the Café Momus.

Recognition and acceptance came to Mürger with the publication of his stories. Victor Hugo was one of his admirers. In collaboration with Théodore Barrière he put together several of his tales into a five-act play, which opened to great success on November 22, 1849, with the title *La Vie de bohème, comédie en cinq actes en prose*. Two years later his stories were compiled and published as a book with the title *Scènes de la bohème*.[1] In subsequent editions, the title was modified to *Scènes de la vie de la bohème*.

Creating a play from Mürger's short stories required limiting the material to be included and developing a plot to carry the narrative forward in an integrated manner. Théodore Barrière, a contemporary playwright whose other work did not achieve lasting prominence, joined Mürger in this effort. Since Rodolphe, the leading man, was to be a poet, Mürger included some of his poetry, and a composer named Pierre Julien Nargeot was enlisted to set the verses to music. The five-act play that emerged was an immediate success.[2]

The play opens with the Bohemians at a garden picnic. Rodolphe joins the group. Thereafter the action moves to the adjoining garret rooms of Rodolphe, Mimi, Marcel, and Musette. Mimi, coughing and obviously suffering from tuberculosis, leaves Rodolphe but later in the play returns to his garret room to die.

Five decades would pass before Puccini's four-act opera *La*

Bohème would open. It was almost immediately popular. The cast of the opera includes the four Bohemians, their names changed to their Italian equivalents: Rodolfo, Mimi, Marcello, and Musetta, as well as Benoît, the landlord. Its action begins in the garret with Rodolfo and Mimi meeting and falling in love. The second act portrays Bohemian life in a plaza in front of the crowded Café Momus. Mimi, having left Rodolfo, returns gravely ill to him in the third act. The final act follows the play closely as Mimi dies of tuberculosis in Rodolfo's garret room.

Now successful, Mürger had become portly and had male-pattern baldness. He no longer lived in a garret. He met Anaïs Latrasse, a young woman with an abusive husband from whom she had separated but had been unable to obtain a divorce. Soon she and Mürger were living together in a loving relationship that would last throughout the remainder of his life. They found a country home outside of Paris. While he continued to write, she opened an antique store that was sufficiently profitable to provide for their needs. In August 1857, Mürger was made a Chevalier of the French Legion of Honor, which brought with the honor not only a red ribbon but also a modest state pension.

Throughout much of his adult life, Mürger was plagued with recurrent bouts of purpura—multiple hemorrhages into the skin. Purpura is often associated with life-threatening bleeding, but this was not the case for Mürger. It did, however, put him in the Hôpital St. Louis on several occasions, once for as long as five months. He attributed this illness to his copious consumption of coffee; there is little reason to think that was actually the cause. In January 1881, he suffered an acute blockage of the artery to his left leg, probably a thrombotic complication of his purpura. Gangrene followed, and he became gravely ill. A priest administered the last rites. Henry Mürger died on January 28, 1861, at the age of thirty-eight.

—

Whereas a romantic view of Marguerite/Violetta's tuberculosis in Dumas's novel and play is never far from the surface, the same is not always true for the illness of Mürger's Mimi. Mimi is a prominent character throughout Mürger's stories. Her name is given as Lucille, a clear reference to Lucille Louvet, one of the three women in Mürger's life who served collectively as a model for Mimi. Tuberculosis took the lives of two of these three *grisettes*. As in life, Rodolphe nicknames Lucille Mimi. One of the stories, *Mademoiselle Mimi*, is devoted to her and presents her as an opportunist, a *grisette* aspiring to life in the *demi-monde*, a fickle and unfaithful lover to Rodolphe. Mimi's death in a hospital is described with resignation and acceptance. Only a few paragraphs are devoted to it. In the opera, however, a more romantic view of tuberculosis and Mimi's death emerges.

In one of Mürger's stories, *Francine's Muff*, a romantic view of tuberculosis is presented, a view carried forward into the play and opera. This tale departs from the model of the others in which Rodolphe and Mimi are the principal characters. In this story their parts are taken by Jacques and Francine—name changes but not material changes in the characters.

> She [Francine] met Jacques, and fell in love with him. Their liaison lasted six months. They met in the spring, they parted in the autumn. Francine was consumptive; she knew it, and her lover Jacques knew it, too. A fortnight after starting to live with the girl, he learnt the truth from a doctor friend of his. "She'll go out with the yellow leaves," the latter had said.[3]

Read in English translation today, Mürger's stories are delightful. They are filled with humor. The craftsmanship of Mürger's writing is impressive. One understands immediately why they were popular when published serially in the 1840s. Converting the short stories, each an independent piece, into a play presented somewhat of a challenge. It is probable that Mürger's collaborator, the playwright Théodore Barrière, had a major role in crafting a plot that would carry the scenes through some sort of logical progression. What emerged was a romantic love story centered on Rodolphe, modeled after Mürger, and a consumptive Mimi, modeled after Mürger's three *grisettes*. Images were taken from various ones used in Mürger's stories. When, in 1896, Giacomo Puccini with librettists Giuseppe Giacosa and Luigi Illica created the ever-popular opera, *La Bohème*, the same plot and incorporated scenes were used. In fact, the modern rock opera *Rent* closely follows much of the same plot, tuberculosis being replaced by AIDS as the pervasive, consuming disease.

The touching scene in which Mimi's candle is extinguished and relit from that of Rodolfo is familiar to every opera lover. It was taken directly from *Francine's Muff*. Mimi drops her key. The two touch hands as they search the floor for the key. Mimi finds it, but pushes it under the bed, assuring that she will not be able to regain her own room and will spend the night with Rodolphe (in the opera, it is Rodolfo who finds the key and pockets it).

In the play, Mimi dies of tuberculosis—she is portrayed as consumptive throughout—and her death is romanticized. That the play ends this way was at the insistence of Barrière; Mürger would have preferred a happier ending. Again, the source is *Francine's Muff*, not *Mademoiselle Mimi*. Francine's hands are cold. Jacques gives her her muff and kisses her as she dies. "Oh, my youth, it is you that is being buried," Rodolphe cries as the play ends.[4] This line is taken directly from *Francine's Muff*, where Jacques is heard to cry it as Francine's coffin is lowered into the grave.

PART III

EBB TIDE

—Retreat to the Mountains—

CHAPTER 8

MAGIC MOUNTAIN

THOMAS MANN, 1875–1955

—Separation—

We practise a pretty high degree of retirement from the world, we up here. No doubt about it.
—Thomas Mann, The Magic Mountain

THOMAS MANN's iconic novel, *The Magic Mountain*, stands as the classic description of life in a tuberculosis sanatorium. Set at the International Sanatorium Berghof in the Swiss Alpine village of Davos, its narrative captures the isolation and the insular self-containment of communities of tuberculosis sanatorium patients. No other work has done this so well.

Paul Thomas Mann—always known as Thomas Mann—was born in the Hanseatic city of Lübeck on the Baltic coast of Germany on June 6, 1875. The Mann family was a prosperous one in Lübeck, a thriving mercantile city at that time. Thomas Mann's father, Thomas Heinrich Johann Mann, was a grain merchant, the third-generation owner of a prosperous family business. His mother, Julia da Silva Bruhns Mann, had been born in Brazil, where her emigrant Lübeck father had married Maria Luiza da Silva, a Portuguese Creole (Creole persons were those of Spanish or Portuguese paternity born in the colonies of the New World). When Julia was seven years old, her mother died, and her father returned to Lübeck, bringing the girl with him.

Mann's boyhood was not unusual for the second son of a late nineteenth-century merchant family in Lübeck. Following primary school he entered the Katharineum in 1889, a secondary school with a greater emphasis on discipline than academic achievement. As a school youth, he began to write poetry and short stories, but his literary efforts were not encouraged by the faculty. He was often melancholy, a forerunner of a hypochondria that would emerge during adulthood. And he developed a homosexual attachment to a younger boy, although it was probably never overtly manifested. In later life he would also sometimes struggle with latent homosexual urges, and homoerotic images would appear in some of his writing.

Life at home was happy for Mann. He was close to his older brother, Heinrich, who also had literary interests. Music played an important role in the home. Mann's mother was musical and he inherited some of her talent. His father shared her interest in music. Mann took violin lessons and played the piano.

In October 1891, when Mann was sixteen, his father died of bladder cancer. His widow, Mann's mother, found herself in a reasonably comfortable but not affluent financial situation. She sold the large Mann family home in Lübeck and retired to a smaller villa in the nearby countryside. A year later she moved with her three younger children to Munich, where her parents lived. Thomas Mann stayed in Lübeck, boarding with one of his teachers. In May of 1893, his first published short story appeared in a literary journal that he started with a friend; the journal managed to print two issues before failing. When he finished school at the Katharineum with a desultory academic record in 1894, he went to Munich to join his family. There he worked in a bank and enrolled in the Technische Hochschule. He continued to write short stories, but had little success in finding publishers for them.

Literary success finally rewarded his persistence and irrepressible creative urge. His short stories were published in literary journals in 1894 and 1896, and in 1897 he was paid 150 marks for a collection of his stories. He felt secure in his aspiration to be an author.

In 1897 Mann conceived of a novel based on his own family history in Lübeck. Originally given the working title *Downhill*, it was to trace the Mann family story over three generations. He adopted the name Buddenbrook for his family, and the novel emerged as *Buddenbrooks*. Five years went into writing this epic novel, and during those years Mann continued to write and publish short stories and novellas. *Buddenbrooks* was published in late 1901. It was an instant success. The first printing of 2,000 copies sold out quickly. Second and third printings of 10,000 and 25,000 copies also sold well. Mann's twenty-percent royalty made him comfortable, and the success of the book established him as an author of note. He spent the summer of 1902 enjoying his success and relaxing at a spa at Mitterbad, probably suffering more from hypochondria and ennui than disease.

In 1901 Mann entered the German army to discharge his obligation of one year's military service. Training consisted largely of parading, and he soon developed a tendinitis in his foot so that he could not march. After a brief hospitalization, he was discharged as unfit.

In Munich, Mann entered into an intellectual circle of writers and artists, frequently attending their salons and gatherings. At one of these he met Katia Pringsheim. She came from a prominent, liberal, intellectual Munich family. Her father was a professor of mathematics. Her mother was an early activist for women's rights. Professor Pringsheim was Jewish. His wife, Katia's mother, was of Jewish heritage, but her family had converted to Christianity two generations earlier. The family was secular and did not practice any religious faith, but Katia's Jewish antecedents would have an impact on the couple and their family when Nazis came to power in Germany. Mann soon began to court Katia, but she initially turned him aside, as she did others who sought her affections. He persisted, and she became more responsive to his suit. On October 3, 1904, they became engaged when, with her assent, he asked her father for her hand. They were married on February 11, 1905.

The young couple found a third-floor apartment in Munich overlooking the park of the Prince William Palace. They were happy there. He wrote, and she assumed the role of business manager for his increasingly successful literary career. Katia became pregnant. Their first child, a daughter, Erika, was born on November 9, 1905. Five more children followed: Klaus, born November 18, 1906;

Angelus Gottfried (called Golo), born March 27, 1909; Monika, born June 7, 1910; Elisabeth, born April 24, 1918; and Michael, born April 21, 1919. The Manns moved to a larger apartment, and summered outside of Munich in Bad Tölz.

Katia's health began to fail. In May 1911 Thomas Mann and Katia went to the Island of Brioni, off the Dalmatian Coast, hoping that she would improve with a rest at the shore. The weather was unpleasant, however, and they moved on to Venice. Katia was plagued with cough and persistent fever. Her doctors told her that she had tuberculosis. In March 1912 Katia went to a sanatorium in Davos, where she would spend the next six months seeking a cure for her tuberculosis. Mann remained in Tölz with their children.

On May 15, 1912, Mann went to Davos to visit his wife, staying there until June 12. While there, in parallel with the narrative of *The Magic Mountain*, he was told he had tuberculosis and should remain as a patient.

> I had been at the so-called Berghof ten days, sitting out on the balcony in cold, damp weather, when I got a troublesome bronchial cold. Two specialists were in the house, the head physician and his assistant, so I took the obvious course of consulting them. I accompanied my wife to the office, she having been summoned to one of her regular examinations. The head doctor...thumped me about and straightway discovered a so-called moist spot in my lung.[1]

Mann ignored the doctor's advice to remain in Davos and returned to his family in Tölz. Katia stayed in Davos for six months. She would have recurrent illness for the next several years.

Mann conceived of *The Magic Mountain* while visiting his wife in Davos. He began work on it the following summer and labored over it intermittently for more than a decade. At various times he published or gave readings of completed chapters separately. The book grew to increasing length before it finally appeared in two volumes on November 28, 1924.

—

The Magic Mountain is an extraordinary work. Monumental in size and scope, it is powerful when read today, and certainly must have been even more so when read in the years following World War I. Superficially, it is the story of Hans Lorenz Castorp who arrives in Davos, Switzerland, to visit his cousin, Joachim Ziemssen at the Berghof Sanatorium, where Joachim is being treated for tuberculosis. While there, Castorp is examined by Hofrat Behrens, the physician-in-chief, and found to have tuberculosis. He is advised to remain at the Berghof, a stay that ultimately stretches into seven years. The plot is slow-moving—tediously so, by the standards of modern fiction—and, in fact, very few events of note transpire. The book is much more than this slow-moving story, however.

The circumstances of Mann's life that led to this work are of interest. The book, at least for the first chapter, is based on Mann's own experience while visiting his wife in Davos. In an afterword written for the Lowe-Porter English translation of *The Magic Mountain*, Mann wrote:

> There is a chapter...where Hans Castorp dines with his cousin Joachim in the sanatorium restaurant, and tastes not only the excellent Berghof cuisine but also the atmosphere of the place and the life "*bei uns hier oben*." If you read that chapter, you will have a fairly accurate picture of our meeting in this sphere and my own strange impressions of it.
>
> The impressions grew stronger and stronger during the three weeks I spent at Davos visiting my wife while she was a patient. They are the same three weeks Hans Castorp originally meant to spend at Davos—though for him they turned into the seven fairy-tale years of his enchanted stay. At least *one* of his experiences is a pretty exact transference to my hero of things that happened to me; I mean the examination of the carefree visitor from the "flatland," and the resulting discovery that he himself is to become a patient too![2]

One can read Mann's work on several levels. It is rich in social commentary, much of it relevant today, even more relevant in the time in which it was written. The importance of love in human relationships is explored. A chapter is devoted to death and its images. Theology is explored; the conflicts between the liberal thinking of Protestantism and conservative tenets of Catholicism or Judaism are played out in a conflict between characters in the novel; their disagreement crests in a duel culminating in the death by suicide of the representative of conservative theologies. A dominant theme in the work is the separation from the real world that life in a sanatorium entailed, and the aura of a special status it accorded to those suffering from tuberculosis.

The novel is rich in imagery, and the principal characters have metaphorical roles. Castorp is clearly an everyman, an ordinary person—an average man, a victim of his circumstances who yields to them with little understanding. Perhaps a Candide, perhaps a Don Quixote. He exercises little independence, and accepts his fate without question. He accepts his place in the society of sufferers at Davos, finds the Berghof a nonthreatening environment, and wishes not to disturb his established life patterns there.

Hofrat Behrens, as the principal doctor, controls absolutely the lives of all of the patients at the sanatorium. The name, Hofrat, can perhaps be translated as a supreme court judge or a high-level advisor. When Castorp is put to bed by Hofrat, the order is described as the edict of "the highest authority in our little world." Only he can tell the sufferer how much disease is present. "One can never know," Joachim tells Castorp, speaking of the patient's dependence on the edicts of the doctor. Hofrat is repeatedly referred to as "the Hofrat" and often as Rhadamanthus, the mythical judge of Hades. Hofrat, with his X-ray machine and his fluoroscope, is able to see deep within those who inhabit the Berghof. As a portraitist, he has exceptional skill at portraying skin, the body's external surface that covers the secrets within. Nothing is unseen by the Hofrat. Hofrat represents incontestable authority, whether civil, religious, or medical.

Castorp befriends an Italian patient named Ludovic Settembrini, whom he calls a humanist organ grinder. A professor before falling ill, Settembrini represents liberalism in the various metaphors of the book. But also an organ grinder, because he interacts with people at an ordinary, nonacademic level. Mynheer Pieter Peeperkorn, a major character in the latter half of the book, clearly represents the coarse materialism of life outside the society of the sanatorium. He is moneyed and self-centered, yet generous. He brings to the Berghof the ways and mores of the flatland, which are portrayed as crude and vulgar. He suffers not only from tuberculosis, but also from malaria and perhaps other ills. He does not survive life at the Berghof.

Perhaps the most complex character in the novel is Clavdia Chauchat. Castorp is taken with her beauty, yet unable to speak to her for nearly a year. Finally, while intoxicated at a Witches Night celebration, he professes his love for her and then becomes her lover for one night before she leaves the sanatorium. That event transpired on February 29, a unique date for events that were at the time and remained unique. Clavdia has a kind but not passionate affection for Castorp. When she finally returns it is in the company of Peeperkorn, whose needs she serves as would a servant or a nurse with kindness and devotion, but not passion. More than any other character in the novel, she represents humanity, humanitarianism, goodness, and the ideals of human being. She is kind and loving to Castorp. She is attentive and dutiful to Peeperkorn.

Acknowledging that *The Magic Mountain* is an onion of a book from which many successive layers can be peeled, it is also a story of persons with tuberculosis in the sanatorium era of the late nineteenth and early twentieth century. No other written work recounts this narrative better. Life in a sanatorium differs from life in "the 'plain'—the 'flatland,' as the healthy normal world was called up here," not only for those at the Berghof, but for those curing from the dread disease in sanatoria throughout the world. Hans Castorp epitomizes those many sufferers. "When, from the point of view of 'those up here,' he considered life as lived down in the flatland, it seemed somehow queer and unnatural."

A dominant theme of *The Magic Mountain* is the separation of the Berghof and its residents from the world below. In Castorp's words,

> We practise a pretty high degree of retirement from the world, we up here. No doubt about it. Five thousand feet up, we lie in these excellent chairs of ours, contemplating

> the world and all that therein is, and having our thoughts about it.[3]

The physical separation determined by geography is accompanied by a cultural and social separation that is even more profound. As Easter approaches,

> The ocean of time, rolling onwards in monotonous rhythm, bore the Easter-tide on its billows. And they observed the season at the Berghof, as they did consistently all the recurrent feasts of the year, by way of breaking up and articulating the long stretches of time. At early breakfast there was a nosegay of violets at each place; at second breakfast each guest had a coloured egg; while sugar and chocolate hares adorned and made festive the midday table.
>
> "Have you ever made a voyage by steamship?"...asked Herr Settembrini strolling up to the cousins' table, toothpick in mouth.... "These rabbits and coloured eggs somehow remind me of the life on board a great ocean-going boat, where you stare at a briny waste and a bare horizon for weeks on end."

When Hans Castorp asks Clavdia Chauchat if she has a postage stamp, she replies she has none.

> Why should I? I never write a letter. To whom should I write? I seldom do, even a card.... I have no one to write to. I have no contact with the flatland, it has fallen away. We have a folk-song that says: "I am lost to the world"—so it is with me.

In fact, Frau Chauchat has a husband from whom she is separated by her illness, not only physically but also in personal terms.

There is an inescapable permanence to the isolation of tuberculosis patients in sanatoria. Their stays seem interminable. Time becomes meaningless.

> To measure one's own private time, that time which for the individual in these parts was so closely bound up with space—that was held to be an occupation only fit for new arrivals and short-termers.... What we spend up here isn't time at all.

Castorp asks about patients being discharged, and his cousin commented "that, so far as he knew,...nobody did leave very much, up here, as a matter of fact." Settembrini tells Castorp of a young man, "a husband and son, who was up here for eleven months.... They let him go home, provisionally, as much improved, he returned to the bosom of his family,...his wife and his mother. The whole day he lay with the thermometer in his mouth, he took no interest in anything else. 'You don't understand,' he said. 'No one understands who has not lived up there. Down here the fundamental conception is lacking.'" And so he returned to the Alpine world he knew.

Castorp's cousin, Joachim Ziemssen, has been a soldier, and he wishes nothing more than to return to his military unit. Against the advice of the Hofrat, he leaves the Berghof with the advent of a new year. He is initially happy and sends cheerful postcards back to Castorp. In April he is promoted to become a lieutenant. Then his health begins to fail, and by summer he is on sick leave. In July he returns to the Berghof. Hofrat "sentence[s him to] four weeks in the 'caboose' [bed rest]." His disease worsens, however, and three months later he dies. Returning to the flatland is not an option consistent with life.

If those with tuberculosis are condemned to live apart from the world below, they are also accorded special status. Hans Castorp assumes the privilege of using the familiar second person form of address to Clavdia Chauchat under circumstances where a closer relationship might normally be required. "Your illness gives you freedom," she notes. There are many rituals that bind the residents of Berghof to one another in this special society. Daily rests at prescribed times in cold mountain air on the balconies of their rooms are ritualized by a formal routine of wrapping the body in blankets and a sleeping bag. Residents "measure" by taking their temperature with a thermometer held beneath the tongue for precisely seven minutes. And they carry, as a badge, a "Blue Peter," a bottle in which they collect their sputum.

The special society of patients at the Berghof has an initiation ritual. It is the examination, not done immediately at entry, but after a probationary period of some weeks during which the novitiate has the opportunity to experience the sanatorium life in all of its aspects and to accept it. This examination is carried out with the patient stripped of his or her clothes and all bodily and personal secrets while the Hofrat thumps on the chest and listens to the novice's respiration with a stethoscope. The physical exam is followed by a radiologic one, both making a glass plate of the image and studying the lungs with a fluoroscope. These images, which expose the interior of the body, become precious marks of acceptance into the Society Berghof. Castorp exchanges his with Clavdia, and keeps hers close to his heart during her absence.

Romantic liaisons develop among the inhabitants of Mann's Berghof, as they did at sanatoria everywhere. Castorp's affair with Clavdia Chauchat is one example, but Mann makes it clear that there are other romantic encounters between the men and women incarcerated in the Alpine retreat. Separated from the real world, these couplings were to be expected.

Ultimately Hans Castorp leaves the Berghof, but not because his disease status has changed. Indeed, Mann makes it clear that Castorp has already improved much earlier and no longer needs therapy at the Alpine retreat; he is simply so established in the community that he cannot separate himself from it. Castorp leaves to join the German army as World War I erupts, just as did young men throughout Europe and, ultimately, America. The reader last sees Castorp struggling through mud as his infantry group charges into battle. Castorp falls face down into the muck. We do not know whether he falls to gunfire or simply stumbles. We do not know if he gets up to continue the senseless charge.

Mann's view of tuberculosis, as reflected in *The Magic Mountain*, is clear. A chronic and often fatal disease that was common in Europe during the years he wrote the book, it gave to its victims a special status. The usual treatment, optimistically called "curing," removes the sufferers to a sanctuary designed to reinforce this special status. In the sanatorium they relinquish much of their individuality and independence of thought to the disease and to "the Hofrat." By thus submitting, they may have hope for relief from their illness. In this enfolding milieu, they are separated from the ordinary, plague-ridden world of the flatland below. Entry into this separated community is via a one-way road; few or none successfully leave. Once having entered into the sanctuary and having been accepted into the special society, there can be no return. Nor is there desire to leave. Only death or a catastrophe of the magnitude of a global war can provide an escape—and that escape is to a dangerous, unknown, and unknowable fate.

Mann himself refused the invitation to enter into the sanctuary. His wife, Katia, submitted. She was fortunate. She was released from the Berghof after six months, but, as Mann worked on his novel, she continued to suffer from tuberculosis relapses and retreated back to Alpine sanctuaries from time to time. That both he and Katia would live for many more tuberculosis-free years Thomas Mann could not have anticipated as he worked on his masterpiece.

—

From 1914 through 1918, Europe was convulsed by World War I. While Mann supported the German position, he was angered by the apparent brutality of German troops in Belgium and the unrestricted German submarine warfare. He was an intellectual and a liberal, more at home in a literary world than a military and political one. He reported for military service, but was rejected as unfit, perhaps because the evaluating officer did not want to induct the now famous author rather than because of Mann's physical state. Mann sold the house at Tölz in July 1917. As had been the four wartime years, the years following the war were difficult ones for Germans. Uncontrolled inflation made day-to-day living difficult for Mann, Katia, and their now six children. Mann was plagued with a variety of neurotic, psychosomatic complaints, but he was physically healthy. If the diagnosis of tuberculosis he was given during his visit to Davos in 1912 was accurate, the disease did not recur during his lifetime. Katia was less fortunate. Illness pursued her intermittently. From February to March 1924, the year in which *The Magic Mountain* was published, she was back in the Swiss Alps nurturing her health, this time at Clavadel, not far from Davos.

Despite Mann's neuroses and hypochondria and despite occasional struggles with his sexual orientation, Mann's life with Katia was a happy and rewarding one. On the occasion of his silver wedding anniversary on February 11, 1930, he wrote:

> Here again I do not know how to thank enough the wife who now for five and twenty years has shared my life—this difficult, so easily tired and distracted life, which asks, above all, for so much patience; I do not know how, without the wise, courageous, delicate yet energetic assistance of my incomparable companion and friend, I should sustain it even as well as I do.[4]

As Germany moved into and through the 1920s, the nation was increasingly troubled with political unrest in the aftermath of the war. Mann stayed apart from it, despite his liberal views and general pride in his German nationality. He was now a famous author and much sought after as a lecturer. Usually accompanied by Katia, he traveled extensively to speak and read from his work. In November 1926 he was elected a Senator of the newly established literary section of the Prussian Academy of Arts.

On November 12, 1929, the Nobel Prize committee of the Swedish Academy telegraphed Mann to advise him that the academy had voted him the Nobel Prize for Literature. Mann and Katia traveled to Stockholm to receive the prize, which was awarded by King Gustav V at a ceremony on December 10. The cash award of 200,000 marks provided welcome assistance in dealing with debts accumulated during the post-war years by him and his children. Many more public appearances followed.

Fame suited Thomas Mann well. He enjoyed the attention it brought him. He continued to write, but spent much of his time and energy traveling and lecturing, often reading from his published and in-process writings. Royalties and speaking fees provided him with a comfortable income.

While Mann's life was serene, if busy, that of the average German was not. The economy of the Weimar Republic floundered, awash in inflation and fiscal chaos. National Socialism—Nazism—was on the rise. Mann was not overly interested in politics, and he was apparently not initially threatened by the Nazis: "a mischief which will soon pass," he commented in an interview. Soon he became concerned and expressed his apprehensions. On October 17, 1930 he spoke out more forcefully, warning against National Socialism. His remarks precipitated a brouhaha in the hall as right-leaning members of the audience protested his remarks. Speaking at a celebration of the four-hundredth anniversary of the founding of the Lübeck Katharenium, his alma mater, on September 4, 1931, he warned against anti-liberal radicalism. He was booed by the students.

On July 31, 1932 the National Socialist (Nazi) party won 230 of 608 seats in the Reichstag. On January 30, 1933 Adolf Hitler became Chancellor of the Reich, displacing from power Paul von Hindenburg, the aging former field marshal and President of the Weimar Republic. On February 27 the Reichstag building burned, its flames probably ignited by Nazis. On March 24, Hitler became dictator.

Accompanied by Katia, Mann was abroad lecturing during those tumultuous months. Yet his anti-Nazi remarks were not unnoticed. His name appeared on a list of those guilty of "intellectual high treason." His daughter called him from Munich and warned him that it was not safe to return to Germany. He went first to Bandol on the French Riviera. His family joined him there. After a number of intervening exile retreats, he and his family settled in German-speaking Switzerland near Zurich in the autumn of 1933.

During the next three years, Mann became an increasingly outspoken critic of Nazism. Originally thinking of himself as not interested in politics, he was a liberal in thought and was repulsed by the totalitarian and anti-Semitic stance of Hitler and his government. He refused membership in the Literary Chamber of the Reich. He remained in exile in Switzerland, but traveled extensively to lecture in Europe and America. In 1935 Harvard University awarded Mann an honorary degree. Ten days later he and Katia dined privately at the White House with President and Mrs. Roosevelt.

Mann's oldest daughter, Erika, an outspoken intellectual and liberal, had her German citizenship revoked in June 1935. Now divorced from her German husband, she married W.H. Auden and became a British citizen. In November of 1936, Mann became a Czech citizen. Two weeks later, the German government revoked his citizenship, an action more provoked by his outspoken anti-Nazi stance than his acceptance of Czech citizenship.

In May of 1938 Thomas Mann established residence and began the process of naturalization in the United States, where he would remain throughout the war and post-war years; he became a citizen in June 1944. He received an honorary degree from Columbia University and accepted an appointment as a lecturer at Princeton University. Additional honorary degrees followed, including ones from Princeton and the University of California at Berkeley. He and Katia rented a house in Princeton. Yale University established a library for his manuscripts and papers. Mann refused an honorary presidency offered to him by the League of American Writers because of the communist orientation of the league. In October 1940 Mann began series of monthly radio broadcasts to Germany on behalf of the allied cause. In 1941 he and Katia built a house in Pacific Palisades, California.

Mann continued to write and lecture. Famous and celebrated, he received many accolades. His writing did not, however, revisit tuberculosis, the topic of *The Magic Mountain*. In 1946 his health began to fail, and he was found to have lung cancer. He underwent a successful removal of part of his right lung and recovered from this setback. In 1952 he returned to live near Zurich in Switzerland. There he died on August 12, 1955 at the age of 80. Katia survived until 1980, remaining in Switzerland, where she died at the age of 96.

CHAPTER 9

STORY TELLER

KATHERINE MANSFIELD, 1888–1923

—*Denial*—

I have been obsessed by the fear of death.

—*Katherine Mansfield,* Journal

THE EARLY years of the twentieth century began with the self-confidant Edwardian era, followed by the seemingly pointless "Great War" that engulfed Europe and America from 1914 to 1918. That era continued with the desperate rush to freedom from all restraint that marked the "roaring twenties." It spawned creativity and originality in artistic and literary arenas that pushed forward boundaries set in earlier, more conservative times. Katherine Mansfield was in the van of creative writers of the time. She died of tuberculosis. As she struggled with illness, she was enormously productive of the short stories that epitomized her literary work. Moreover, she wrote letters and kept a journal that have survived. Most notably, she wrote short stories that challenged readers' intellects. She did not incorporate her illness directly into her literary work, but some of her fiction certainly reflected her failing health.

The third child of Harold and Annie Dyer Beauchamp, Katherine Mansfield was born in Wellington, New Zealand, on October 14, 1888. Her parents named her Kathleen Mansfield Beauchamp; later she adopted the name Katherine Mansfield, by which she was always known. Not pretty, pouty-faced, stammering, she was an unhappy schoolchild in Wellington. She was often rebellious and nonconforming. Her father was domineering and distant, her mother chronically ill. The family was wealthy and socially prominent in New Zealand.

At the Wellington Girls' High School, Katherine Mansfield began to display her nascent literary talents, publishing a short story and receiving prizes in French and English. She also developed her first close friendships, one of which, with a Maori girl named Maata Mahupuka, evolved into the first of a number of intimate sexual relationships with women. As a twelve-year-old she met Arnold Trowell, a child-prodigy cellist, with whom she would develop her first heterosexual love. She herself studied the cello and became accomplished with the instrument.

In January 1903 the Beauchamp family sailed to England, where Katherine enrolled in Queen's College, London. Trowell was in London at the time, and she saw him frequently, but he did not respond to her as she hoped he might. He did, however, open her eyes to a world of art, music, and literature that had not been available to her in New Zealand. Late in 1906 she returned to New Zealand. She was unhappy there, and was uncomfortable in the social circle of her family. July 1908 found her aboard the *S.S. Papanui*, gladly returning to London.

Mansfield's return was not as happy as she had anticipated. At best, her first year in Europe was tumultuous. She was chronically short of money—throughout much of her life her wealthy father rejected her pleas for support—and earned small sums as a bit-part actress. Arnold Trowell spurned her. She responded by shifting her affections to Arnold's twin brother, Garnet, also a musician, albeit not as accomplished as his brother. Soon she and Garnet, whom she probably seduced to initiate their relationship, were lovers, and she became pregnant. She also established a lesbian relationship with Ida Baker, who would be her companion through much of the illness-plagued later years of her life.

During the winter months, Mansfield met George Bowden, a singer. He became enamored of her. She sought security and a father for her unborn child. They were married on March 2, 1909. Their marriage was not consummated, and within a week she had left him. They would live together from time to time over the next two years, but they never established a true marital relationship. Years later, they divorced so that they could each remarry. She briefly resumed her relationship with Garnet Trowell, and then took refuge at a spa in Germany. In June 1909 Katherine Mansfield gave birth to a premature, stillborn infant.

During this unhappy period Katherine Mansfield matured into the woman she would be throughout the remainder of her Bohemian life. As Hans Christian Andersen's ugly duckling became a swan, so she became a beautiful, talented, literate, witty young woman. She was described by an acquaintance as "extremely attractive—the dark lively intelligent face under the dark fringe."[1] Eccentric, certainly; impetuous, often; creative, always; Katherine Mansfield joined the circle of European literary giants who lived free-will, Bohemian lives during the first two decades of the twentieth century. D.H. Lawrence, who would also succumb to tuberculosis, became a close friend. So also did Virginia Woolf and Aldous Huxley. She began publishing the short stories upon which her literary reputation would be built.

In December 1911 Mansfield met John Middleton Murry at a party. Murry was the editor of *Rhythm*, a literary journal in which one of her stories had been published. They began corresponding, and in April she invited him to move into her apartment, although he was to occupy a separate bedroom. Platonic relationships were inimical to Katherine Mansfield, however, and within a few weeks the two were sharing the same bed. She joined him in editing *Rhythm*, and continued to write well-received short stories. Albeit occasionally stormy, the relationship between the two lasted and, for the most part if not entirely, was characterized by fidelity. Murry was an inept lover, however. Katherine very much wanted children, but she had become barren, probably as a result of gonorrhea. On May 3, 1920, the couple were married, four days after finalizing her divorce from Bowden.

In July of 1912, Katherine Mansfield developed pleurisy. She traveled to Belgium and Switzerland and recovered her health. This episode probably marked the onset of the tuberculosis that would recur and then plague her for the last decade of her life.

The next several years were generally happy, although often impoverished, years for Mansfield and Murry. They both pursued their literary endeavors with increasing success. They socialized with the European literary world. With the outbreak of war in 1914, Leslie Beauchamp, Katherine's younger brother, enlisted in the British army, only to be killed by an exploding grenade in Belgium. Murry and Mansfield journeyed to southern France in November 1915, staying in Bandol, a small fishing village on the Mediterranean Coast east of Marseille. Murry returned to London in December. In the spring of 1916 he took a civilian position with the British Intelligence Service. He was successful in this position and increasingly occupied with it, thus further distancing him from Katherine during their intermittently interrupted domestic relationship and marriage.

In April 1914 Katherine Mansfield again suffered from pleurisy, likely a further manifestation of her nascent tuberculosis. In January 1915 she suffered a respiratory infection with an annoying cough, probably the onset of the pulmonary tuberculosis that was soon to erupt. And erupt it did. In November 1917, she had an episode of fever accompanied by chest pain. Her doctor advised her once again to travel to southern France, and so she returned to Bandol. The journey exhausted her, and she was slow to recover her strength. In February she wrote in her journal:

> What happens is that I come in absolutely exhausted, lie down, sit up and sit in a daze of fatigue—a horrible state—until 7 o'clock. I can barely walk—can't think, don't dare to go to sleep because if I do I know I'll lie awake through the night, and that is my horror.... The pain continues in my left shoulder.[2]

The shoulder pain she described may have been a recurrence of her pleurisy or it may have been a manifestation of active tuberculosis in the upper part of her left lung. On February 19, 1918 she experienced her first substantial hemorrhage from tuberculosis.

> *February 19.* I woke up early this morning and when I opened the shutters the full round sun was just risen. I began to repeat that verse of Shakespeare's: "Lo, here the gentle lark weary of rest," and bounded back into bed. The

> bound made me cough—I spat—it tasted strange—it was bright red blood. Since then I've gone on spitting each time I cough a little more. Oh, yes, of course I am frightened. But for two reasons only. I don't want to be ill, I mean "seriously," away from J. J. is the first thought. 2nd, I don't want to find this is real consumption, perhaps it's going to gallop—who knows?—and I shan't have my work written. That's what matters. How unbearable it would be to die—leave "scraps," "bits"...nothing real finished.[3]

From this time forward, Katherine Mansfield would never be free of tuberculosis and the mental anguish as well as physical suffering that it brought her. The disease would dominate her life until it finally claimed her.

Katherine Mansfield spent the winter of 1920-21 in Menton on the French Riviera, close to the Italian border. A medical report from a Dr. Bouchage, who cared for her at that time, provides the only surviving description of the extent of her disease.

> When I first saw her, Oct 15 1920, she had been suffering from lung troubles for three years, and was at the time complaining of bad attacks of coughing, especially morning and evening (in spite of codeine taken 6 times a day for the last two years),...[and] of palpitations in the heart on the least provocation. (Digitalis mixture taken for 6 months previously).
>
> Previous history. Age 32. Excellent health till 20. Married for the 1st time at 18. Had 2 years after an attack of peritonitis (very likely from gonococcal origin) [with] white [vaginal] discharge for 4 months. Left salpinx was removed then. Since that time she has never been quite well....
>
> During the war, exertions and worries. In autumn 1917 actual disease began and since then has been more or less an invalid with lungs and heart and rheumatic troubles. No T.B. in family history.
>
> In 1919 Dr. [Victor] Sorapure in London found "practi-

> cally the whole left lung and the right apex full of large and moist rales." Since I have attended Mrs. Murry...there have been variations in the condition. At first I found the area described in the left lung posteriorly with moist rales and also rales of a finer character in left apex front and back and a few dry noises at right apex posteriorly. In November this condition was improving very satisfactorily. In December condition gradually got worse after mental exertion and worries, and the heart, which had only been showing signs of tachycardia, began to be very troublesome.... A gland on the right side of the neck grew...and had to be punctured twice lately, in March. The cough has been very distressing at times. Expectoration has increased in quantity, and examination (microscopical: guinea-pig inoculation) has shown tubercular bacillus.[4]

This description makes it clear that Mansfield had far-advanced, cavitary disease, and a modern medical reader immediately assumes that in the absence of effective treatment her disease would ultimately claim her life. She was repeatedly advised to seek care in a tuberculosis sanatorium, which she did not—could not—do. In fact, the physician whom she most trusted, Victor Sorapure, advised against sanatorium care. In October 1918, Mansfield wrote from Hampstead to her husband (whom she affectionately called "Jack") in London:

> My dear Jack,
> I confess that these last days my fight with the enemy has been so hard that I just laid down my weapons and ran away, and consented to what has always seemed to me the final intolerable thing, i.e. to go into a sanatorium.
>
> Today, finally think it over, and in view of the fact that it is not, after all, so much a question of climate as of regime... I am determined by my own will, to live the sanatorium life *here.*[5]

There follows a list of items for this regime, concluding with:

> (7) I shall not worry.
>
> You see, Jack, for the first time, today I am determined to get well.... I am going through with this and I want you to help me.... [6]

Throughout her illness, Mansfield continued to write, and her writing seemed to sustain her. In her journal one reads:

> *June 10* [1919]. I have discovered that I cannot burn the candle at one end and write a book with the other.
>
> Life without *work*—I would commit suicide. Therefore work is more important than life.[7]

Despair and anger gave way at times to resignation. On December 15, 1919, the suffering woman wrote:

> All these two years I have been obsessed by the fear of death. This grew and grew and grew gigantic, and this it was that made me cling so, I think. Then days ago it went, I care not more. It leaves me perfectly cold.... Life either stays or goes.[8]

Later in the same month:

> Surely I do know more than other people: I have suffered more, and endured more. I know how they long to be happy, and how precious is an atmosphere that is loving, a *climate* that is not frightening. Why do I not try to bear this in mind, and try to cultivate my garden?[9]

Not willing to enter a sanatorium, Mansfield did embrace the popular idea that certain climates were salubrious for those who suffered from tuberculosis. As had Percy Bysshe Shelley and John Keats, she chose to go to Italy for the winter of 1919-20. From the time of her first hemorrhage that so closely paralleled Keats's experience, she had been fascinated by an idea that her disease closely resembled that of the poet whom she so admired. Mansfield went to San Remo on the Italian Riviera, not distant from Menton in France, where she would also seek a milder climate the following two winters. The Alps of Switzerland had acquired a substantial reputation as favorable places to "cure," and sanatoria were proliferating there. In May of 1921 she made her first trip to Switzerland. She spent much of the next year and one-half in the Valois region of the Rhone River valley.

Mansfield's letters to her husband from San Remo reveal desperation, a hope for recovery that she must have known was baseless, a rejection of the inevitable—denial. On November 8, 1919, she wrote:

> You see, I *am* getting better; my body is getting better. I have a theory that perhaps the creaking and pain I had were caused by the moist spot drying up in my bad lung. It's quite possible.[10]

Three days later she wrote:

> I have just had the extraordinary comfort of seeing a really first-chop doctor—the man Ansaldi.... It was getting dusky. There was a ring at the bell and I opened the door and nearly fell into the arms of a beaming, glistening Jewish gentleman mit a vite felt hat. I immediately decided he was a body-snatcher and said, most rudely, "Vous désirez?" At which he replied "Ansaldi" and abashed me very much. He came in—dark bright skin, gleaming eyes, a slight stoop....
>
> My bad lung he says is drying: there's only a small spot left at the apex. (When I was in London there was a spot the size of a hand.) The other has also a small spot at the apex. I told him my history to date and he says that I have gained weight and can eat are excellent signs. There is no reason (bar accident) why I should not recover. "Never to be a lion or shoot the chamois or the hare"—*figurez-vous*, my darling, I'd rather feed them with rose leaves—but to lead a normal life, not the life of an invalid. The chances, he says, 99 to 100 that I can do this.

Was Ansaldi a quack intent on deceiving her to gain her confidence and enrich his purse? Probably not. One must recall the famous French aphorism, "to cure sometimes, to relieve often, but to comfort always." He most likely thought that his patient would die soon and that comfort, even false hope, would benefit her more than a realistic prognosis. Thus, he supported her denial. One must also note that assessment of the extent of tuberculous lesions in the lung by physical examination is difficult, at best. X-ray examination of the chest was available at this time in some medical facilities, but none of the doctors Mansfield consulted appear to have used this modality. In fact, it is not evident that Mansfield ever had a radiologic examination.

Back in Menton the following year, her daily letters to her husband once again reveal a desperate longing for the recovery she must have realized would never come. On September 16, 1920 she wrote:

> I'm better today, fever gone, but weak as a butterfly and *thin* as a match.

The following day:

> Dearest, I'm better. Temperature normal—pain gone—up and lying in the salon. I am eating again too and now really *will* mend. But I have never been so thin—not even in Paris. I simply melted like a candle with that fever.

And on September 19;

> Your Wig is still so weak that she can't walk straight—sometimes I fling myself at the doors or take a great high step in the air. But I *am* really on the mend, and as to my cough—fancy, I've been here five days and I hardly cough at all. This morning in fact I didn't cough at all and can't remember if I have until now, 6 P.M. I have only to get my strength back after this "attack."

Two days later:

> I wish I were stronger. I'm so much better. My cough is nearly gone. It's nothing but *de la faiblesse* and I know it will pass.

These excerpts from her letters epitomize both the longing for recovery and the denial of her disease progression that characterized her attitude towards the disease and the feelings of many other victims of tuberculosis. To accept a slow and relentless progression to death was impossible. Thus every small sign of improvement from day to day or even hour to hour was seized as a token of healing, evanescent as such small changes inevitably proved to be. Hope, always hope, even in the face of apparent hopelessness.

Although rejecting sanatoria, Mansfield did not reject treatment of her disease. Indeed, she embarked on a variety of therapies that had little benefit and in some instances probably did her harm. In 1919 she received a series of antiserum injections, which made her ill. In the first half of 1922 she put herself under the care of Ivan Manoukhin, a Russian doctor who had worked at the Pasteur Institute in Paris before the war and had been head of an infectious disease hospital in Kiev during the war. He had opened a clinic in Paris where he was treating patients with tuberculosis by X-irradiating their spleens. The modern medical reader must immediately suppose that this therapy could be of no benefit and might weaken the body's innate defense mechanisms against tuberculosis. In Mansfield's case, the treatment caused radiation sickness and appeared to have little effect on the course of her tuberculosis. At a later date she was treated in the loft of a cattle barn where she inhaled the breath of cows. Bizarre as these therapies sound, they were not unusual for the time.

Mansfield's published stories did not deal with her illness. Nor did she tell of the lives of other ill persons or write specifically about tuberculosis. One of her best known stories, "The Fly," was written in 1920 while she was in Switzerland. A parable, it surely contains a metaphor for her tuberculosis, but it is a much more complex an allegory than simply that.[11]

The story opens as old Mr. Woodifield—a name borrowed from a fellow victim of tuberculosis whom she had met in Switzerland, and perhaps also echoing her birth name of Beauchamp—meets "the boss." Mr. Woodifield, Mansfield tells us, "clings to [his] last pleasures as the tree clings to its last leaves." Thus do tuberculosis patients savor their few joyful moments.

The narrative shifts as Mr. Woodifield leaves, and the boss grieves over the loss of his only son who was killed six years earlier on the battlefield of the Great War. "'My son!' groaned the boss." Does the boss represent God, whose only son, Jesus, died in the service of humanity? Mansfield was not religious, and it is not credible to attribute such a Christian interpretation to her. Perhaps the boss represents impersonal fate or destiny. The son may harken back to Mansfield's brother, who was killed during the war. Thus, we are led to contrast his noble death with the impending tortured end of her life.

The narrative then shifts to the fate of a fly, and the fly most certainly represents Mansfield, herself, as she battles her inescapable, fatal destiny—an insect, struggling fruitlessly against the inevitable.

> At that moment the boss noticed that a fly had fallen into his broad inkpot, and was trying feebly but desperately to clamber out again. Help! help! said those struggling legs. But the sides of the inkpot were wet and slippery; it fell back again and began to swim. The boss took up a pen, picked the fly out of the ink, and shook it on to a piece of blotting-paper. For a fraction of a second it lay still on the dark patch that oozed round it. Then the front legs waved, took hold, and, pulling its small sodden body up it began the immense task of cleaning the ink from its wings. Over and under, over and under, went a leg along a wing, as the stone goes over and under the scythe. Then there was a pause, while the fly, seeming to stand on the tips of its toes, tried to expand first one wing and then the other. It succeeded at last, and, sitting

> down, it began, like a minute cat, to clean its face. Now one could imagine that the little front legs rubbed against each other lightly, joyfully. The horrible danger was over; it had escaped; it was ready for life again.
>
> But just then the boss had an idea. He plunged his pen back into the ink, leaned his thick wrist on the blotting paper, and as the fly tried its wings down came a great heavy blot. What would it make of that? What indeed! The little beggar seemed absolutely cowed, stunned, and afraid to move because of what would happen next. But then, as if painfully, it dragged itself forward. The front legs waved, caught hold, and, more slowly this time, the task began from the beginning.
>
> He's a plucky little devil, thought the boss, and he felt a real admiration for the fly's courage. That was the way to tackle things; that was the right spirit. Never say die; it was only a question of.... But the fly had again finished its laborious task, and the boss had just time to refill his pen, to shake fair and square on the new-cleaned body yet another dark drop. What about it this time? A painful moment of suspense followed. But behold, the front legs were again waving; the boss felt a rush of relief. He leaned over the fly and said to it tenderly, "You artful little b...." And he actually had the brilliant notion of breathing on it to help the drying process. All the same, there was something timid and weak about its efforts now, and the boss decided that this time should be the last, as he dipped the pen into the inkpot.
>
> It was. The last blot on the soaked blotting-paper, and the draggled fly lay in it and did not stir. The back legs were stuck to the body; the front legs were not to be seen.
>
> "Come on," said the boss. "Look sharp!" And he stirred it with his pen—in vain. Nothing happened or was likely to happen. The fly was dead.

The narrative ends in emphasizing the absence of concern that impersonal fate has for its victims.

> The boss lifted the corpse on the end of the paper-knife and flung it into the waste-paper basket.
>
> "Bring me some fresh blotting-paper," he said, sternly, "and look sharp about it." And...he fell to wondering what it was he had been thinking about before. What was it? It was.... He took out his handkerchief and passed it inside his collar. For the life of him he could not remember.

Impersonal fate cares not for the life of Katherine Mansfield.

Although Mansfield despaired of any hope for cure, she was not ready to submit completely to the Captain of Death. Futility, hopelessness, these are attitudes towards one's future that only deeply depressed persons can sustain. Mansfield was not ready to give up trying, hoping, grasping for life even as she, indeed, gasped for breath.

In 1914 George Ivanovich Gurdjieff, a Russian Armenian, opened an Institute for the Harmonious Development of Man in Moscow. He left Russia following the revolution there, and in 1922 re-established himself and his institute at *La Prieuré de Basses-Loges* in Fontainebleau, south of Paris. The regimen that he instituted there was a tightly controlled one that included communal living with assigned chores and total submission to his dicta. Ill and not far from death but still not abandoning hope, Katherine Mansfield entered the Spartan quarters of his institution on October 16, 1922. Before leaving Switzerland she had apparently set aside her denial and faced the reality of impending death sufficiently to have written a will.

At Fontainebleau she was too weak to participate in most of the activities of the institute, although she did help in the kitchen. Submission was a dominant theme of Gurdjieff's program, and Mansfield submitted not only to his program but also to her disease. At the same time, she felt she was improving—denying her obviously advancing state of decline. She asked Murry to join her, which he did. Upon his arrival on the evening of January 23, 1923, she ran up a flight of stairs to show him her room. At the top she began to cough and then to bleed fatally from her lung, coughing up copious amounts of bright blood. And thus her life ended, ebbing with a massive pulmonary hemorrhage.

Katherine Mansfield was a literary genius whose life was taken prematurely by tuberculosis. Her letters told of the suffering, the hopelessness, and the denial with which she viewed her condition. Although she did not write directly of her disease in her stories, Mansfield's "The Fly" certainly represents the absolute despair with which the young author viewed her unremitting illness. She, the fly, immersed in disease, the ink, was at the mercy of impersonal fate or a malevolent God, the boss, in whom she professed not to believe. Doctors of the time, who prescribed their nostrums and dispatched victims of tuberculosis to sanatoria, led sufferers to believe there might be hope. Mansfield might hope, but she knew there was no escape for her. Her only recourse was to deny the gravity of her illness.

CHAPTER 10

ARISTOCRAT

W. SOMERSET MAUGHAM, 1874–1965

—*Hope*—

I suppose it depends on how much you value life.
—*W. Somerset Maugham,* Sanatorium

W. Somerset Maugham was an enormously successful author. Urbane and made wealthy by royalties from his writing, he was a prototypic product of the Edwardian age. He traveled extensively and drew many of the plots for his writings from his travels. A homosexual with many male lovers, he also enjoyed heterosexual love. He suffered from recurrent episodes of tuberculosis, and incorporated his sanatorium experiences into a short story.

Maugham was born on January 25, 1874 in Paris, France, where his parents were members of the British expatriate community. His mother died of tuberculosis when he was eight years old; his father died of cancer two years later. He then went to England, to the small town of Whitstable near Coventry in Kent, to live with an uncle who was a church parson in the small town. His inheritance was paltry, nor was his uncle prosperous, and Maugham would know privation during his adolescence. In England, struggling with a new language, he developed a stammer that plagued him during his long life whenever he was under stress.

Maugham was initially schooled in Whitstable, but then sent to King's School in Canterbury. He was called Willie by his family, schoolmates, and later by his adult friends. One of his classmates was named Leonard Ashenden. Maugham used minimally altered names of his friends in his fiction, and Willie Ashenden would become the protagonist or narrator of many of his stories.

Maugham's schooling was interrupted in 1888 when he developed pleurisy, almost certainly the onset of the tuberculosis that would recur during his adult life. He went to Hyères on the French Riviera, where the benign climate might prove salubrious, and spent the winter there. He returned to Kent in the spring, but the following winter found him back in Hyères, again seeking better health. He did not return to King's School, but went to Germany, where he spent a year studying at the University of Heidelberg.

Maugham returned from Germany to enter medical school at St. Thomas' Hospital in London. He spent five years studying medicine, the later years on clinical services. For a time he seemed bent on a career in obstetrics, but this calling faded as did his entire interest in medicine. While a medical student he began writing short stories and determined to make his way as an author. He produced his first novel, *Liza of Lambeth*, which was published in 1897. It sold out its first printing of 2,000 copies within a few weeks. He passed his medical licensing examination in October 1897 and was offered an obstetrics post at St. Thomas' Hospital. He turned it down. Maugham would never enter the practice of medicine.

Excited by the success of his first novel and with his head full of ideas for further literary efforts, Maugham traveled to Italy. For the next four decades he traveled to many parts of the globe, always writing, always finding plots during his travels for his stories, novels, and plays. Some of his best known tales had their genesis in the South Pacific. Increasingly prosperous, he returned to England or France to live an aristocratic life of luxurious leisure, but always with morning hours devoted to writing. His way of life was the antithesis of the Bohemian life styles of Henry Mürger and Katherine Mansfield.

When World War I erupted in Europe, Maugham was too old and too short of stature for military service. He volunteered to go to France with the Red Cross. His intent was to serve as a translator, for he was bilingual in French and English and fluent in German. He soon found himself in field hospitals, using his surgical skills to dress wounds and treat war casualties. In the World War I battle zone of Flanders he met Gerald Haxton, who would become his friend, companion, secretary, and the most enduring among his homosexual partners. Maugham's battlefield service was interrupted when he was asked to go to Switzerland with the British intelligence service. This he did, later using his experiences there to write spy stories. Subsequently he traveled to Petrograd (Leningrad, St. Petersburg), then the capital of Russia, on another intelligence mission. He traveled by ship from London to Tokyo, and then reached his destination via railroad across Siberia, returning to London via Norway and Scotland.

Maugham was an active homosexual. His first such liaison occurred while a student at Heidelberg. Many others, including that with Haxton, followed. He also had heterosexual affairs. In April 1906, he met and fell deeply in love with Sue Arthur Jones, recently divorced and an actress in one of his plays. They were soon bed partners. He purchased a wedding ring, sailed to New York, where she was appearing in one of his plays, proposed to her, and invited her to accompany him to Tahiti. She spurned him, however, later to marry a British earl. He was more successful in suit of Syrie Wellcome, whom he first met at a London party in 1913. A year later the pair were lovers. She was the estranged wife of American pharmaceutical executive Harry Wellcome, who had refused her a divorce. Wanting a child, she became pregnant by Maugham, only to miscarry. Once again pregnant, she underwent a Caesarian section to deliver a daughter, Liza, on September 1, 1915. Maugham found himself ambivalent about his paternity. He left Syrie and their daughter to travel to the South Pacific, finding stories there and writing. Upon return he found Syrie now free from her husband. They were married before a judge in New Jersey on May 26, 1917. Although the marriage would last for ten years before ending in divorce, Maugham vacillated in his feelings for Syrie, and they often lived apart.

In his later years, Maugham lived alone in London or in his mansion on the Riviera. He entertained frequently. He wrote only occasionally. He played bridge, often at his London club, the Garrick Club. He died on December 15, 1965, one month shy of his ninety-second birthday.

Tuberculosis was a recurrent visitor to Maugham. Perhaps infected by his mother, he developed tuberculous pleurisy as a student, but recovered his health. While in Switzerland on his espionage assignment, he relapsed and became ill with pulmonary tuberculosis. He was not hospitalized at that time, but did return to England. When he was asked to go to Russia in 1917, he consulted a doctor who told him that the trip would not help his health. On the other hand, the physician averred, his trip would be patriotic and would help the war effort. Back in England after the arduous journey with his tuberculosis again symptomatic, he was advised to go to a sanatorium. The popular cure sites in Switzerland were inaccessible because of the war, and so he went to a sanatorium in Banchory, near Aberdeen in Scotland. After six weeks of bed rest, he was allowed up, and when the summer of 1918 arrived, he and Syrie rented a house in Surrey. The following winter found him once again hospitalized in Banchory. Improved again and hopeful of continued good health, he and Syrie spent the following summer in a house at Banchory. Thereafter he remained well except for a six-week period in a sanatorium in Java.

—

Maugham wrote while resting for his tuberculosis. His novel *The Moon and Sixpence* was written at such a time. Subsequently he wrote a short story called "Sanatorium," which clearly reflects his personal experiences as a patient with tuberculosis.[1] It reveals his perceptions of the disease. It provides a more accurate account of sanatorium life than does Mann's *The Magic Mountain*. It is a complex story, revealing much about those who take refuge from the world in sanatoria. All of the varied disease perceptions and individual responses to them are illustrated in the characters of Maugham's story.

Ashenden, Maugham's protagonist, is ill with tuberculosis. Like Maugham's, his circumstances do not permit a retreat to Switzerland, so he goes to a sanatorium in Scotland. Maugham's story describes the daily routines of life at the sanatorium. The characters are richly drawn. As initially seen, they are all submissive and passively accepting of that which life has dealt them. They see themselves as having no other option.

Sanatorium life is sheltered. Many, in fact, most, tuberculosis patients spend years "curing" there. They become dependent upon the shelter provided by the sanatorium.

> They don't want to go. They've been here so long...they can't cope with the outside world. Campbell went away for a couple of months' holiday some years ago. He came back after a week; said he couldn't stand the racket, and the sight of so many people on the street.

There is an element of guilt associated with tuberculosis. Others are not afflicted, so the sufferer inevitably wonders what he or she has done to bring on the inescapable disease.

> Henry Chester was born and bred to lead an average life, exposed to the normal vicissitudes of existence, and when an unforeseeable accident befell him he had no means of coping with it. He was like a brick made to take its place with a million others in a huge factory, but by chance with a flaw in it so that it is inadequate to its purpose. And the brick too, if it had a mind, might cry: What have I done that I cannot fulfill my modest end, but must be taken away from all these other bricks that support me and thrown on the dust-heap?

The response to tuberculosis is necessarily acceptance—submission—although people may deal with this differently, some meekly, some rebelliously. In the end, however, there is no escape and no alternative to resignation. For many, death will be inevitable and unavoidable. Denial is a normal response of many victims, and it allows the victims of tuberculosis to face daily life with some measure of hope, with a positive outlook, albeit perhaps unwarranted.

> Of all those people in the sanatorium he was...the only one who genuinely accepted the inevitable with unconcern. He snapped his fingers in the face of death, and you could choose whether to call his levity unbecoming or his insouciance gallant.

Many of the episodes in Maugham's short story are metaphorical. Two men with advanced tuberculosis who are long-time residents and who are angry rivals in many aspects of sanatorium life find themselves opponents in a bridge game. Each holds good cards, and they bid against one another, finally reaching grand slam, doubled, redoubled, the highest level a bridge contract can reach. Maugham was an excellent bridge player, and the tenseness of this contract is clearly described. Two finesses were required, "and they both came off." But true victory is impossible in the face of the Captain of Death.

> "Grand slam doubled and redoubled. I've wanted to get it all my life and now I've got it. By God. By God."
>
> He gasped. He staggered forward and fell across the table. A stream of blood poured from his mouth. The doctor was sent for. Attendants came. He was dead.

An act of rebellion inevitably causes worsening of tuberculosis, even death. Patients have no realistic recourse but submission. They must never undertake risky activities. Yet, some patients choose to ignore medical advice, hoping to live a fuller life.

> "I wonder if it's worth it. I wonder if it's not better to have one's fling and take the consequences."
>
> "I suppose it depends on how much you value life."
>
> "But is this life?"

Maugham's story concludes by recounting two marriages. One of long standing is disrupted when the husband comes to the sanatorium with tuberculosis. Guilt-ridden, he spurns his wife and puts an end to her weekly visits. The second culminates the romance of two ill patients who marry despite the doctor's warning that doing so will shorten their lives.

> "Do you know what I've done?" asked Templeton. "I've asked Ivy to marry me."
>
> Ashenden was startled.

"What did she say/"

"Bless her little heart, she said it was the most ridiculous idea she'd ever heard in her life and I was crazy to think of such a thing."

"You must admit she was right."

"Quite. But she is going to marry me."

The obvious happiness of the couple influences others and makes them think about the values that sanatorium life has set upon them.

In an ultimate statement of resignation to his disease and yet also rebellion, the tuberculous husband who has spurned his healthy wife—banished her from visiting him, in fact—says to her, "I don't think death's very important, not so important as love." The ultimate irony, perhaps, is hope for love and happiness when death is inevitable.

CHAPTER 11

CHAMPION

ALICE MARBLE, 1913–1990

—*Rebellion*—

I was tired of people telling me what I couldn't do.... I'm never going to get well here.

—*Alice Marble,* Courting Danger

ALICE MARBLE was a remarkable woman. Stricken with tuberculosis, she conquered her disease to continue her domination of women's tennis with championship after championship. She did so after storming out of the sanatorium to which she had been confined. Anger and rebellion were her responses to her illness.

Alice Marble was born in September 1913 in Beckwourth, California, high in the Sierra Nevada Mountains. When she was five years old, she moved with her family to a house on Twelfth Avenue, in the Sunset District of San Francisco. Her father died following an automobile accident two years later. Too young to go to work to help support the family, as did two of her older brothers, she continued in school, where she excelled. Her native intelligence was helped by an exceptional, photographic memory that made studying easy for her. A tomboy and blessed with superior eye-hand coordination, she loved sports. Baseball was her first love, and soon she was pitching balls to players on a semi-pro team, the San Francisco Seals, including Joe DiMaggio. At age thirteen she became the team's mascot. During her first year in high school, her brother gave her a tennis racquet, and she began playing with a schoolmate at nearby Golden Gate Park. Marble's baseball days were over; tennis became her passion. At age seventeen she became the junior champion of Northern California. Her tennis career was launched.

The following summer Marble, now the reigning woman's tennis player of the West Coast, made her debut at the United States Lawn Tennis Association's championship tournament at Forest Hills. It was her first experience playing on a grass-surfaced court, and she lost miserably in the first round of the singles tournament. Paired with Bonnie Miller, also from California, she and Miller won the women's doubles championship. She was back the following year, this time catching the eye of newspaper sports writers, who recognized her innate talent. So also did the well-known tennis coach Eleanor "Teach" Tennant of Beverly Hills, California, who would become not only her coach, but her personal mentor and close friend, both on and off the tennis court. Under her guidance Marble refined her game and went from one championship to the next.

Californian Tennant was a favorite coach of Hollywood movie actors. She coached them at their clubs and on their private courts. She also traveled to William Randolph Hearst's mountaintop estate, San Simeon. Tennant took Marble with her to Hearst's luxurious estate, where she found herself in the company of the era's reigning movie stars, all eager to play with her. Intelligent and a blue-eyed, blond beauty with a lovely, athletic figure—a reporter writing about her compared her to Venus de Milo—Marble enjoyed her time at San Simeon, which stretched to an entire month. Thereafter, she became Hearst's frequent guest, playing tennis during the day and partying with famous guests in the evening. In her autobiography, she recounts an encounter as dinner partner with George Bernard Shaw. Marble had written a high school paper on Shaw, and called upon her memory of his works.

> "What did you talk about?" Teach asked later.
>
> "Him.... I knew the names and characters of every one of his plays, so I talked about his work and he talked about himself. He was a delightful old coot, but so egoistical!"[1]

More championships followed, and in 1934 Alice Marble joined other leading American women tennis players to represent the United States in the Wightman Cup tournament at the famous Wimbledon courts in England. First, however, the Americans were to play in France. On May 1, she and her teammates set sail for Europe. The passage across the Atlantic should have been enjoyable, but Marble felt tired and unwell. In Paris she looked ill to her teammates during practice games, and a French doctor saw her. He found her anemic, but fit to play. During her first tournament match, she played poorly, struggling, losing, and collapsing near the end of the first set. She was carried from the court, unconscious, and taken to the American Hospital at Neuilly. Her chest hurt with every breath. The attending doctor told her she had anemia and pleurisy. Two days later, the doctor told her she had tuberculosis. "I'm sorry, but you will never be strong enough to play tennis again."

After six weeks in the hospital, she was allowed to sail for home. During the first three days of her return passage, the ship's doctor confined her to her cabin; subsequently he allowed her on deck. Teach Tennant met her in New York and drove her across the country to the Pottenger Sanatorium in Monrovia, California. Francis Marion Pottenger, M.D., owned the sanatorium and cared for the patients hospitalized there. Fifty years old at the time of Marble's hospitalization, he had received his medical degree from the University of Minnesota in 1913. He had a national reputation in the field of tuberculosis and had served in leadership positions in many professional societies, including as president of the American Trudeau Society (now the American Thoracic Society), the leading professional society for physicians specializing in pulmonary disease. In 1948 he authored a leading textbook devoted to tuberculosis. His sanatorium was highly regarded.

Pottenger prescribed bed rest for Alice Marble, allowing her up only to use the bathroom, and confined her to her cottage. His initial prescription was for six weeks of rest. As Marble recalled her experience as a sanatorium patient,

> The place was deadly dull, filled with people like me, vegetating.
>
> Dr Pottinger [*sic*] examined me once a week, always with the same comment. "Hm, yes, you're doing nicely."

> "But am I getting well?" I growled. "How's my blood count? How do my lungs look?" I wanted to know specifics, but his replies, always placating, said nothing. I was no longer in pain, but the inactivity was making me weak. I watched the muscles in my arms go slack and my thighs turn to flab. I was watching my body die.

At the end of six weeks, Pottenger told her she needed another six weeks of rest. A fellow patient commented, "They tell everybody they'll be out in six weeks. I've been here two years. You'll never get out."

Marble's account may be flawed—she consistently misspelled Pottenger's name as Pottinger, for example—for it was written more than five decades after the fact. However, if one looks at what Pottenger has to say about treating patients with tuberculosis, one finds in his book an emphasis on bed rest.

> Granting that the patient is properly nourished, rest is the most important single remedy that is employed in the treatment of active tuberculosis. With it properly applied at the right time, most other accepted measures may be applied in a half-hearted manner and still a great proportion of patients will recover; while without it, other measures may be correctly applied and still the great majority of patients will fail to recover.... If each patient is taught how to take proper advantage of rest, he will be put in the way of receiving the greatest possible good from any general plan of treatment adopted.[2]

Pottenger wrote his text, it should be noted, before any effective drug therapy for tuberculosis became available.

Diet was an important part of the treatment of persons suffering from tuberculosis in sanatoria. Pottenger devoted a chapter of his text to it and gave specific details of the menus served his patients. The Pottenger Sanatorium fed patients a 3,400-calories-per-day, protein-rich diet. Such a diet is appropriate for an active, competitive athlete. It is perhaps twice what an average adult at rest requires. Alice Marble gained forty pounds.

Six weeks after six weeks stretched to eight months. Marble's reaction was initially despair, but increasingly anger and rebellion.

> Every day was a slice of hell, and the nights were worse—sleepless, desolate hours of staring into the darkness. I had stacks of books and magazines, but found myself reading the same sentence over and over, with no comprehension. I've always loved to sing, but the words of my favorite songs just wouldn't come.
>
> I begged Pottinger [*sic*] to let me walk in the gardens, but he forbade any physical exertion. Exertion! I had never been bedridden before, never been sick really.... I cried for hours at a time."

In his book, Pottenger includes a three-paragraph section on the "Psychology of the Tuberculous Patient." In fact, even in this brief section, he says little on the subject. His emphasis is on "regulating the life of the patient...in order to make it possible for the patient to cooperate in treatment."[3] One must wonder how much effort in this direction he expended on Alice Marble during his once-weekly visits. Certain it is, however, that his medical beliefs dictated physician control of the patient's body and mind.

Then Marble's life changed. One autumn day she received a letter that inspired her to take control of her life away from Pottenger and those who felt she should be consigned to a lifetime of illness.

> Dear Alice,
>
> You don't know me, but your tennis teacher is also my teacher, and she has told me all about you. Once I thought I had a great career in front of me, just like you thought you had. Then one day I was in a terrible automobile accident. For six months I lay on a hospital bed, just like you are today. Doctors told me I was through, but then I began to

> think I had nothing to lose by fighting, so I began to fight. Well, I proved the doctors wrong. I made my career come true, just as you can—if you'll fight. If I can do it, so can you.

The letter came from Carole Lombard, whom Alice Marble had never met. Lombard's "terrible auto accident" had disfigured her famously glamorous face, and she underwent extensive plastic surgical procedures to restore her beauty. Teach Tennant gave tennis lessons to Lombard, and encouraged the movie actress to write the supporting—and challenging—letter to Marble during her confinement to the Pottenger Sanatorium. About six months later the two famous women, both of modest family backgrounds, met, and they became close friends.

On an October day not long after she received the Lombard letter, Alice Marble had her bags packed when Teach Tennant arrived to visit. She walked out of her cottage and into Tennant's car. Her sanatorium stay was over. Tennant was sympathetic; Marble later quoted her as saying about Pottenger:

> That son of a bitch Pottinger [*sic*].... He's been stringing me along, taking my money, and doing nothing to make you better. I could have kept you in bed and stuffed you with food!

Tennant's criticism, if accurately quoted, has to be put in medical context of the time. Pottenger's treatment in his sanatorium did not differ from the standard treatment for persons afflicted with the disease. Sanatorium care and a regimen of rest were felt by nearly all medical authorities to be essential for recovery from tuberculosis.

Tennant did not keep Marble in bed and stuff her with food. She put her on a diet. She allowed her up and encouraged her to take walks; the first tour around the block proved to be an ordeal. Gradually, she lost weight and regained some strength. Tennant took her to see a number of prominent physicians, all of whom concurred with Pottenger and suggested she return to his sanatorium. That was not an option in the minds of the two women.

At the urging of Carole Lombard, Marble consulted Dr. Ernest L. Commons in Los Angeles. Commons was a sixty-year-old physician who had graduated from the Medical College of Indiana in Indianapolis and who practiced in an office at 523 West Sixth Street in Los Angeles as a general medical family doctor. Although he had no particular training or expertise in tuberculosis, that disease was well known to all doctors in the 1930s.

Commons listened to her story, examined her, and obtained X-ray images. He told her that she showed evidence of having had pleurisy, and that her lungs had scars of tuberculosis. But he found no indication of active disease. Commons encouraged her to begin a program of increasing activity, and under his guidance and the watchful eye of Tennant, she did so. On a spring day half a year after leaving the sanatorium, Marble stepped onto a tennis court, racquet in hand, to play three games of a set of doubles. That was all that Tennant allowed her on that first day. As the weeks passed, she played more and more tennis, and at the end of the summer she entered her first come-back tournament at the Palm Springs Racquet Club. In the final round, she defeated her opponent in two sets, 6–2, 6–2. She went on to win the California women's title equally handily. The summer of 1936 found Marble back at Forest Hills, where she won the 1936 United States Lawn Tennis Association women's national championship. Tuberculosis would never again limit this champion.

As competing players enter the stadium to take their places at Forest Hills, they pass under an arch upon which are engraved the famous lines from Rudyard Kipling's poem, "If."

If you can meet with Triumph and Disaster
And treat those two imposters just the same

More tournaments followed. Marble won some, lost others, but when concentrating on her game she was unbeatable. At Wimbledon she reached the semifinals in women's singles play in 1937 and 1938 and won the tournament in 1939, the last year it was held before World War II suspended competition there. In the United States, she won singles matches at Forest Hills in 1938 and 1939. In 1940 she crowned her amateur career with "triple crown" victories at Forest Hills in women's singles, women's doubles, and mixed doubles play. At the end of the 1940 season she gave up amateur play to "turn pro" and tour on the circuit of professional exhibition competitions.

In 1938 Alice Marble escaped from Wimbledon to Le Tourquet, a French casino and resort. There she met Swiss banking scion Hans Steinmetz. She fell in love with him immediately, and within a few days after meeting him was making love to him on the beach. Day after idyllic day the couple spent together, followed by romantic nights together. The affair lasted only a week, but she was ready to quit tennis to follow her lover. Alice proposed to give up tennis for Hans. Teach Tennant would have none of this. In the end, Steinmetz ended the affair, bidding Marble goodbye and telling her to return to her career on the tennis courts.

In 1940, with the entry of the United States into war looming, Marble tried to enlist in the WACs (Women's Army Corps). She was turned down as unfit! Army regulations prohibited military service for those with a history of tuberculosis. However, the FBI asked her to act as a spy; that is, to report on seditious comments she heard during her travels. She did report on a number of conversations in Spain, although she thought the content was innocuous.

During the war years Marble joined with other professional tennis players to play exhibition matches at army bases—more than 500 of them. In 1941, at the Stage Door Canteen in New York City, she met Captain Joseph Crowley, an Army Air Corps pilot and intelligence officer. Three months later they were engaged. Their lives were often separate, he away on military missions, she on exhibition tours. But in 1942 they were married, and thereafter they managed from time to time to be together. In 1944 Marble, then five months pregnant and excited about becoming a mother, was in an automobile accident and sustained major injuries. She survived, but her unborn child did not. Slowly she recovered, and on Christmas Day was celebrating quietly with friends when tragedy visited her again. A telegram brought the news that Joe had been killed in action when his plane was shot down over Germany. She was devastated. She attempted suicide. She withdrew into a shuttered world of grief.

In January of 1942, Marble's close friend, Carole Lombard, had been killed in an airplane crash. Clark Gable, her husband and also a close friend of Marble, had been devastated, but eventually pulled himself out of the depression that followed. In early 1945 he sent three dozen red roses to Marble. The card that came with them said, "If I can do it, so can you." Those words echoed the note from Carole Lombard that had induced Marble to leave the tuberculosis sanatorium. Once again, they turned her around.

Marble had barely emerged from the seclusion of her grief when she was approached by an army intelligence officer. She was asked to become a spy—to return to Switzerland for the purpose of stealing the Nazi bank records held by Hans Steinmetz, her former lover. She accepted the challenge, received intensive training, and then was flown to neutral Switzerland to conduct tennis clinics and play in exhibition matches. As expected, Steinmetz sought her out. Alice Marble found herself disconcertedly attracted to him. In fact, resumption of their intense romantic relationship brought joy to her. Yet she put her feelings aside, managed entry to Steinmetz's vault, and then was shot by a double agent during a harrowing escape. Rescued by an American intelligence officer, she recovered in a Swiss hospital. Her efforts succeeded in uncovering the financial plundering of many prominent Nazis. Steinmetz cooperated with the now victorious allies, and the banking data was used at the International Military Tribunal in Nuremberg that convicted Nazi leaders.

With the end of the war and Marble back in California, one might have expected a return to her former professional tennis career. That did not happen. Asserting the independence that her marriage and adventures as a spy had given her, she broke with Teach Tennant. It was an acrimonious ending to a long relationship. Tennant went on to coach other rising tennis champions. Marble also taught and coached. She died on December 13, 1990 at age 77.

CHAPTER 12

THE RACK

DEREK LINDSAY, ~1920–2001

—*Desperation*—

> *The damned disgrace is to pay lip service to a whole system of treatment which doesn't repay its existence by its results.*
>
> —*Derek Lindsay,* The Rack

ONCE IN A while a rookie baseball player comes to bat for the first time in his first major league game and hits a home run. Not often—only a bit more than two dozen times in American baseball history. English author Derek Lindsay, writing under the *nom de plume* of A.E. Ellis, achieved the literary parallel of a first-time-at-bat home run with his 1958 novel, *The Rack.*[1] Promoted with an enthusiastic blurb by Graham Greene, the book became a best-seller and a Book of the Month Club selection in the United States. Following that astounding entry into the world of authorship, Lindsay's literary career ended. He published nothing more. He was himself a victim of tuberculosis, and much of his novel is autobiographical.

Lindsay was orphaned at the age of three and raised by an aunt. He had little contact with other children. He served in the British army during World War II as a captain, although he saw little actual warfare. Following the war he attended Oxford University. While a student he published a short story, apparently his only other published work. His studies were interrupted by tuberculosis, and he went to a sanatorium in the Alps seeking a cure. As a result of his disease he underwent surgical procedures that left him with only one functioning lung, his other lung, a diseased lung, lost perhaps to surgical removal or perhaps to collapse by thoracoplasty. Thereafter he was treated with drugs and remained healthy, but reclusive and troubled by psychological demons. He wrote a play, *Grand Manoeuvres*, based on the life of French army officer Alfred Dreyfus; it was produced at London's National Theater, but closed after a short run. Lindsay died in July 2001, hit by a bus while crossing a street in London.

—

The Rack is set in the fictional town of Brisset, high in the Alps of the French department of Haute-Savoie, nestled, perhaps, on the lap of Mont Blanc, the highest of Europe's Alps. It is a town of sanatoria and pensions housing tuberculous consumptives.

> They varied from large modern buildings to chalets on the wooden façades of which were painted: "*Sanitorium-Pension. Bons Soins. Tout Comfort. Cuisine Soignée. Prix Très Modérées.*" They were everywhere, on all levels, clustered as tightly and haphazardly as booths on a fair-ground.[2]

A few skiers make their way to Brisset, but they are outnumbered by the many sufferers seeking cures from tuberculosis.

> They were of all ages, though the young predominated.... Young girls,...young men,...the pears or peaches of a dishonest fruit vendor, resplendent without and rotten within.

It was November late in the 1940s, a time when the sanatorium movement was at its acme, a time when rest dominated the treatment of tuberculosis, a time when collapse therapies—pneumothoraces and thoracoplasties—were employed to put individual lobes of lungs at rest and to close cavities, a time when newly discovered drugs for tuberculosis were but dawning faintly on a distant horizon. It was a time when the advances in treatment of tuberculosis that would make it no longer a dread disease loomed but had not yet arrived.

Paul Devanant, Lindsay's twenty-seven-year-old protagonist, has spent the previous two years as a student at Cambridge University. He was an infantry captain during the World War II. During the time since his discharge he has been ill, increasingly so, with one futile medical evaluation after another until his diagnosis of tuberculosis was finally made. With five other student sufferers sponsored by the International Student Organization, abbreviated ISO, he is headed for a three-month stay at a sanatorium in Brisset named Les Alpes, "indistinguishable in appearance from the type of large continental hotel constructed at the turn of the century." There they would soon be joined by similar ISO-sponsored students from other European countries. Paul Devanant is the oldest and also the sickest member of the British group.

The journey by train up to the mountain haven, the entry into the sanatorium for a proposed limited but eventually prolonged stay, the dictatorial nature of the medical staff, and the description of the first meal all evoke images of Thomas Mann's classic work, *The Magic Mountain*. Lindsay certainly intends the reader to make this comparison. Yet, *The Rack* is profoundly different from its literary predecessors. *The Magic Mountain* and Maugham's *Sanatorium* are works that are set in tuberculosis sanatoria. They recount life in these institutions. Many of the events and daily activities described, including those that surprise the modern reader, represent sanatorium life reasonably faithfully. However, the main thrusts of Mann's and Maugham's writings are portrayals of the complex interactions of the people in the closed and remote sanatorium environment. Allegorical meaning is readily recognized in the players and their roles in the drama that unfolds. Tuberculosis and the treatment prescribed for it are incidental to the narrative. In Lindsay's book the opposite is generally true. While the flow of the narrative builds upon activities of and interactions among the students at the sanatorium, for the most part they are incidental to the story. The focus of *The Rack* is on the ominous, relentless progression of Devanant's disease and on the repeated frustrations of sufferers at the inefficacy of treatments given. Detailed and medically accurate descriptions of the therapeutic interventions to which he is subjected are interwoven with equally detailed descriptions of the complications that follow. Paul Devanant's tortuous course is reminiscent of the torture of the innocent insect described in tuberculosis-afflicted author Katherine Mansfield's short story, "The Fly."[3]

Upon arrival, the ISO-sponsored students are assigned to double rooms on the upper floors; a small number of private patients are housed in larger rooms on the lower floors. Paul Devanant is assigned to share a room with John Cotterell, an Oxford University student whom he befriended on the journey from England. During the initial evaluation, Paul is found to be sputum-positive, that is, to have tubercle bacilli evident in his sputum. He is thus considered infectious. All of the other British students are sputum-negative. As a result, John Cotterell is reassigned to another room, and a Polish student with long-standing disease, Kubahskoi, becomes John's new roommate. The initial X-ray studies also reveal that Paul is sicker than his other compatriots, and he is confined to his bed and room.

Following their initial medical evaluations, the British students compare notes. Paul, although the sickest, is the most naive, this being his first hospitalization for tuberculosis. The students are skeptical of the benefits of many treatments commonly offered. "The damned disgrace is to pay lip service to a whole system of treatment which doesn't repay its existence by its results," comments one student bitterly. "Why...should we expect to overcome it by suppressing symptoms?" To that, another replies, "The question is, Man having fallen, what methods have you to substitute for the treatment which you find so unsatisfactory?" In this section of the novel, author Lindsay displays a remarkably detailed and accurate knowledge of then current modalities of treatment, drawn, one must believe, from his own experience with the dread disease.

Life for the students at Les Alpes is a constant battle with the penurious administrators and the authoritarian physicians, who seem more interested in preserving the wealth of their sanatorium employment than the health of their sanatorium patients. Many of the battles focus on the food served to them, which is poor in both quantity and quality. Protests are mounted, sometimes erupting into violence, but little changes.

At the end of three months, the prescribed time having elapsed, the British students are expected to return to England. Four of them do so, but Paul Devanant and John Cotterell are considered too ill to be discharged. Paul's life becomes one of unremitting tedium, punctuated by compulsive taking of and recording his temperature and collecting his expectorated sputum in a "hygienically sealed...blue container." He is confined to his bed and room. There is no evident potential denouement. He questions his friend, John Cotterell, who has experienced previous tuberculosis sanatorium sojourns.

> "You told me last night that you had already spent six months in a sanatorium."
>
> John Cotterell laughed. "Six months with this illness is not a very long time."
>
> "It isn't! Then how long do you think I will be here?"
>
> "I'm afraid it's very difficult to say."
>
> "But how long could it be," insisted Paul.
>
> "There isn't really a time limit. It all depends on what happens."

Through the remainder of the narrative, *The Rack* recounts the agonizing vicissitudes of the life of a tuberculosis sufferer.

> Some of these students had been imprisoned in concentration camps; the conditions in which they had lived had induced T.B. of the bone or of the lung, sometimes both. One form of imprisonment had been exchanged for another; where they had been confined to cells, they were now confined to beds, where they had lain in fetters, they now lay in plaster casts. They had previously existed in daily dread of summary death; it was now only the method, not the threat which had altered.

Not day by day, not week by week, but month by month Paul's condition changes, sometimes improving, sometimes relapsing. And the life stories of other patients at Les Alpes are similar, sometimes tragic. John Cotterell succumbs. A desperate young woman who is dying of the disease leaps to her death from the balcony outside the window of her room.

Over time, Paul is destined to improve, to be allowed up and into the village, only to relapse. This course is repeated over and again during two years in Brisset. All new therapies provided but short benefit. When the improvement that came with bed rest is followed by relapse, Paul is offered pneumothorax, a procedure designed to put a lung at rest and to collapse its upper portions. It is in these upper segments that tuberculous cavities in which tubercle bacilli proliferate usually form, and these cavities could sometimes be closed by a pneumothorax.

To induce a pneumothorax, a needle was introduced between the ribs, and air was pumped into the pleural space between the lung and the chest wall to compress the lung. When all went well, the procedure was beneficial. It was especially useful in closing cavities, thus rendering patients noninfectious. However, all did not always go well, and if there were scar-related adhesions between the lung surface and the inner surface of the chest wall, then the lung could not collapse. A remedy often undertaken was cutting these adhesions. A thoracoscope (a metal tube) was introduced between the ribs, and through it the surgeon attempted to cut away the scar tissue preventing lung collapse. Paul Devanant's lung does not collapse, and so he is subjected to thoracoscopy, and with that procedure collapse is achieved. Much-feared complications of pneumothorax and especially of thoracoscopy were exudation of fluid into the pleural space leading to more adhesions; bleeding from the cut surfaces of the adhesions, which could be difficult to control; and infection of the pleural space. If the opening required to insert the thoracoscope permitted the entry of bacteria, then infection of the space—empyema, in medical terminology—resulted.

Paul suffers all of the potential set-backs that sometimes resulted from pneumothorax and thoracoscopy. He requires transfusions from a donor for the bleeding. Managing the infection proves to be a prolonged and difficult battle. In the pre-antibiotic era in which *The Rack* is set, the treatment of empyema was a horrendous torture. Fluid and pus were drained and various antiseptics introduced. Paul Devanant suffers greatly from these complications and therapies.

However, despite the adverse consequences of the intervention, he does improve, only to relapse again.

As patients struggle in their battles against disease, so also the various sanatoria in Brisset struggle to survive on limited financial resources. Those that take ISO students, including Les Alpes, are especially hard-pressed, for the ISO does not pay the full rate. Ultimately Les Alpes closes, and Paul Devanant finds himself seeking another refuge. He finds a pension on the outskirts of the village. There he does well for a considerable period before relapsing again and returning to the then reopened Les Alpes.

Drugs for treating tuberculosis arrive during Paul's stay in Brisset, and he receives them. Streptomycin and para-amino salicylic acid (PAS) are given to him, first one, then the other. In addition, they are instilled into his pleural cavity after it becomes evident that he has not only an empyema caused by the entry of pus-causing bacteria, but also that his tuberculosis had spread to this space. With each of these drugs, he improves. However, his tubercle bacilli develop resistance to each of them, as often happened when drugs were used singly, as they commonly were at that time. He worsens. Hope of drug-induced cure disappears.

When all other measures seem to have failed, Paul Devanant's doctors raise the possibility of thoracoplasty to him. In this procedure, posterior portions of ribs were removed to achieve permanent collapse of the underlying lung. Thoracoplasty required major surgery and was often poorly tolerated by sick patients. It required general anesthesia and surgery with the patient on his or her side with the diseased lung uppermost and the healthy lung beneath it. A major and often life-threatening complication was the spread of disease during surgery from the cavity-laden tuberculous lung to the healthy lung on the other side. Thoracoplasty was first employed in Switzerland in 1885; it was initially met with medical skepticism and caution. However, during the 1930s it came into wider use as thoracic surgeons gained competence with it. Thoracoplasty was not undertaken lightly, and it invoked dread in patients for whom it was recommended. Paul Devanant is terrified of the prospect of this operation—justifiably so.

In reading Lindsay's descriptions of the treatments used for tuberculosis, one cannot but be impressed with the detailed and accurate knowledge displayed by the author. This is true not only for his accounts of sanatorium life and the daily routines of these institutions. It is also true for his descriptions of medical procedures for the diagnosis, evaluation, and treatment of tuberculosis during the sanatorium era. One must suppose that Lindsay's personal experience with the dread disease included not only sanatorium care but also pneumothorax, perhaps also with its complications, and thoracoplasty. The descriptions of drug therapy are somewhat less complete. It is likely that Lindsay's sanatorium treatment, like that of his protagonist, came at a time before the advent in the 1950s of curative drug treatment regimens for tuberculosis.

While the characters in Lindsay's narrative are less important than the disease that dominates their lives, there is one person who enters Paul's life to whom much more than casual meaning may be attached. Lindsay divided his novel into three parts, and in the first chapter of Part II, Michèle Duchesne enters the story. Michèle and health become inescapably entwined in Lindsay's account of Paul Devanant's life. When she is present, he seems to make progress in his cure; when she leaves, the remission fades into relapse.

It is August, nine months after Paul's arrival in Brisset, and Paul is about to be told that his condition is now stable and that he will soon be able to return to England. On the way to this eventful appointment with the doctor, he encounters Michèle.

> At the entrance to the *Service Médical*, sitting negligently in the wheel-chair in which often he had been a passenger, was a young girl so lovely that her presence illuminated the corner of the obscure passage: a very new, cherry-coloured dressing-gown covered with light polka dots, a pyjama jacket open at the neck revealing a cool, white throat. She smiled, got up from the chair and walked over to the lift....
>
> Paul learned that the girl's name was Michèle Duchesne, that she was Belgian, that she was only seventeen years old, and that her room was two doors along from his own on the same floor. One afternoon he encountered her in the corridor, they both stopped, and he asked whether he

> might visit her that evening. Smiling, she assented. And so, after dinner, carrying a box of chocolate cats' tongues under his arm, he knocked on her door.
>
> Wearing an open-necked shirt and white linen trousers, she was sitting cross-legged on top of a heap of pillows at the head of her bed. Shyly she extended a hand of welcome.

Youthful, pretty, gay, flirtatious, Michèle stands in contrast to the other inhabitants of Les Alpes, albeit she also is ill with tuberculosis. Her condition is serious, and she, like Paul, undergoes pneumothorax and thoracoscopy to cut adhesions, but without the complications that Paul suffers. She is at Les Alpes as a private patient, and it strains the finances of her parents in Liège to pay for her care. Many of the sanatorium's patients are attracted to her, but it soon is Paul to whom she becomes attached, first as a friend, then as a lover, then as his fiancée. They plan marriage as soon as they both might escape from Brisset and their illnesses.

Michèle enters into Paul's life at a time when relative health has been restored to him. His diseased lung, collapsed beneath the pneumothorax, is in stable condition, although the pneumothorax will have to be maintained for an additional six years. He should be able to return to England soon and resume his university studies the next year. Not wanting to leave Michèle, he decides to prolong his stay in Brisset. At just this time, Les Alpes closes, and Paul moves into the pension he has found near the village. During the interlude that Paul passes in the pension, Michèle is housed in another sanatorium, the Universel. He visits her there, and she makes frequent visits to Paul's pension chamber. Relative health returns to both of them during the winter months.

As Easter approaches, Michèle makes plans to return to her family in Liège for ten days. Paul and Michèle walk in the wood while waiting for her train.

> Suddenly they came out of the wood into a clearing. Like banks of seats in an antique theatre which had been constructed with the Arve valley as its stage, row upon row of tombstones rose above and fell below the path, covering

> whole acres of the mountainside.... So it was here, discreetly beyond the range of any but the best walkers, that they were accommodated, the former comrades.

This passage describing the cemetery can only be read as presaging relapse for Paul.

Michèle returns from her short visit at her home, and the couple are soon planning marriage. Paul is to go to Liège with her in summer. They make train reservations. But bad news hits them. Paul learns that his sputum is again positive for tubercle bacilli, strongly so.

> The door opened. "*Monsieur*, I am sorry to tell you..." The doctor paused. Paul leant back against the wall. "I am sorry to tell you that your analysis is positive."
>
> "Thank you. Thank you for finding out."
>
> "I am sorry."
>
> "Am I very positive?"
>
> "Very positive."

He returns to Michèle, who is waiting at the pension, to tell her he cannot go to Liège with her. As he enters the room and turns on the light, the bulb explodes, leaving them in darkness. Mme. Anniette, the pension owner, arrives with a flashlight.

> "You are not superstitious, monsieur," she said....
>
> "No."
>
> "Then thank God for it." She crossed herself. "The last time I saw a bulb burst like that, my sister was found hanging from the ceiling of her bedroom."

Michèle departs. She will not return. She is better. Her family is incurring debt and can no longer afford to maintain her in Brisset. Paul resumes his cure, changes doctors, and finds himself once again being invaded by needles and tubes in hopes of dealing with the ongoing infection in his pleural space. Part II of *The Rack* closes with Paul once again ill, feverish, sweating profusely, wracked in a tortured dream.

The hope for health that Michèle brought in Part II left with her. Michèle—goddess of health and well-being—is gone; health is gone. In Part III, Paul finds himself back in the once-again-reopened Les Alpes. He has changed doctors to a physician with a more optimistic outlook for Paul. That does not last, however, as the new caregiver suffers a heart attack and dies, leaving Paul in the care of those who treated him previously. His tubercle bacilli become resistant not only to PAS but also to streptomycin. With no apparent end to his misery, Paul contemplates suicide, and begins to hoard sleeping pills.

Christmas approaches, and on December 23, Michèle appears in his room for a surprise visit. The couple is happily reunited, if only for a short time. And suddenly more good news arrives. Laboratory reports on Paul's pleural fluid show no tubercle bacilli. The good news is short-lived, however, for Michèle has to return to Belgium. Soon thereafter Paul's fevered illness returns. Michelle and Paul's well-being have departed together. His doctors recommend a thoracoplasty, which Paul views as a desperate measure unlikely to offer hope. Paul attempts suicide with his store of sleeping capsules, but bungles the attempt, losing his drugs onto the floor and attracting the unwelcome attention of the staff.

Paul's downward spiral towards doom progresses. The final chapter of *The Rack* describes a world of hopelessness. Word arrived that ISO will no longer support his stay in Brisset; he must necessarily return to England. His doctor argues that his condition will probably be stable.

> "My sanatorium days will be over."
>
> "Precisely. Oh, don't misunderstand me. I'm not saying that you'll be fit enough to compete in next year's Channel swim—neither next year's nor the year after's. But a quiet, reasonable life—that will certainly be possible."

A famous Swiss specialist visits Les Alpes, and Paul arranges for a consultation. After a more thorough examination than the sanatorium doctors have rendered, the visiting professor offers a gloomy prognosis. His pleural space could be managed by a permanent drain or by a thoracoplasty, but neither would prove satisfactory. What Paul needs is to have the lung and diseased pleura removed by a thoracic surgeon. Such major operations are now possible, as antibiotics have reduced the risk of postoperative infections. However, Paul's other lung is sufficiently diseased with drug-resistant tubercle bacilli to make that an unsatisfactory option. The consultant's conclusion is that perhaps all options might be reconsidered after a year or eighteen months of bed rest. Meanwhile, nothing more can be done.

A letter from Michèle's mother arrives while he is seeing the visiting consultant. He opens it upon returning to his room to find that it urges him to give up Michèle, as he has no prospect of offering her happiness.

> "If you love her, as I believe you do, you will see where your duty lies."
>
> "It alters nothing," he told himself. Why did he feel such an intensification of grief? "Nothing is altered," he repeated, half aloud. He covered his eyes with his hand. "Stretch me no more on this rough world." The phrase came irresistibly to his mind.

Paul Devanant picks up his copy of the published journal of Benjamin Robert Haydon, the poverty-stricken, depressed, nineteenth-century English painter and author who committed suicide. There in the final entry he finds it.

> "22nd. God forgive me. Amen.
> Finis
> of
> B.R. Haydon
> 'Stretch me no more on this rough world'—Lear."

> Something was grotesquely wrong. He opened his Shakespeare. "O let him pass! He hates him that would upon the rack of this tough world stretch him out longer."[4]
>
> "The rack," he murmured. "Haydon forgot the rack."

> And his mind still exercised by the strangeness of the omission, he stared across at the half-open window.

With those lines, Lindsay closes his narrative.

—

One cannot follow the relationships of Paul with his disease and of Paul with Michèle without being struck by the parallels they display. Michèle is youthful, pretty, gay. She flirts with the male patients. Although afflicted with tuberculosis, her course is more benign than that of Paul. She improves in Brisset. When Paul meets Michèle his health also improves. At one point Paul wonders to himself, "Could it be that now we are both better we no longer need each other?"

When Michèle leaves, Paul worsens; she represents health and hope, and as she fades from Paul's horizon, so also do they. This cycle is repeated as Michèle returns at Christmas. He is offered some hope, for his pleural fluid does not contain tubercle bacilli and a study in which methylene blue was injected into his pleural space reveals no open connection into his lung. The good news is evanescent, however, for Paul remains ill as Michèle departs for Belgium. When she can no longer return to his life and when there remains no hope of further treatment—these two ominous judgments having been rendered simultaneously—desperation inescapably replaces hope. Paul turns to the window. Perhaps the window looks out on a wintery mountain scene stretching on eternally without end. Perhaps the window recalls the patient who jumped to her death shortly after Paul's original entry into Les Alpes.

—

Sanatoria and the treatment provided at them offered hope to tuberculosis patients. Not all were helped, but many were, and undertaking the cure regimens sanatoria offered meant doing something rather than passively accepting the ravages of the Captain of Death. In fact, while most patients with minimal disease did well at tuberculosis sanatoria, those who had more extensive disease had more guarded prognoses. Of those with moderately advanced disease—Paul's likely state at entry to Les Alpes and probably also that of author Derek Lindsay when he entered an Alpine sanatorium—nearly one in four would ultimately die of tuberculosis.

Paul Devanant and the other students in Brisset went to the mountains with hope. Their hope was hope such as that held by Katia Mann and W. Somerset Maugham as they sought healing in mountainous venues. That Paul's experience was ultimately devoid of hope and akin to the torture inflicted by the turns of a medieval rack was not unique, however. For those with more extensive disease, the "rack of this tough world" was the torture meted out to its victims by the dread disease. Not everyone, and not Paul Devanant, could be helped. For those unfortunate ones, hope yielded to unending anguish and desperation. Only death could ultimately relieve the torture.

PART IV

NEAP TIDE

—Cure—

CHAPTER 13

MODERN POET

SYLVIA PLATH, 1932–1963

—*Ignorance*—

I had very little knowledge about TB.
—*Sylvia Plath,* The Bell Jar

SYLVIA PLATH was born in Jamaica Plain outside of Boston on October 27, 1932, the elder of two children of Otto Plath and his wife Aurelia Schober Plath. Following Otto Plath's death when Sylvia was eight years old, the Schobers (Aurelia's parents) and the Plaths combined their households. Aurelia began teaching, first at local high schools, then at Boston University. In 1942 the family moved to Wellesley, southwest of Boston, a move motivated in part by a desire to be near to the Norton family. Aurelia Plath had become a close friend of Mildred Norton, who also taught at Boston University. The Nortons had three boys, and Sylvia and her younger brother, Warren, frequently played together with the Norton boys. Sylvia attended Wellesley High School (then Gamaliel Bradford High School), where she was an honors student. As a high school student, she dated Perry Norton, the middle of the three Norton boys and her age contemporary. She blossomed as a talented wordsmith, with short stories published in *Seventeen*, *The Christian Science Monitor*, and *The Boston Globe*.

In 1950 Plath entered Smith College. She worked hard and excelled as a student. Her literary horizons widened, and she began to write both poetry and prose. Her social life was that of most 1950s middle-class college women. She dated a number of her male peers, including Perry Norton. In the winter of her freshman year, Dick (Richard) Norton, the oldest of the Norton boys, invited her to the

Yale Junior Prom. That event inaugurated a dating relationship that would last for the next several years, often stormily, often evocative of conflicts for Sylvia over her future. Norton was an honors student at Yale, elected to Phi Beta Kappa, active in intramural sports, and a member of Yale's marching band. He graduated from Yale in June 1951 and entered Harvard Medical School in the fall of that year. After the end of his first year of medical studies, he developed tuberculosis and went to Ray Brook Sanatorium in Saranac Lake, New York for treatment. He would ultimately return to Harvard Medical School to graduate with the M.D. degree in 1957, two years behind his entering class.

Sylvia and Dick Norton exchanged letters, and she visited him at Ray Brook during her Christmas vacation, a visit urged upon her by her mother. Plath's diary entries at that time reveal more about her preoccupation with her own sexuality and depressive feelings than her increasingly complex relationship with Dick. It is clear from these entries that she was not worried about his disease. She wrote about it in matter-of-fact tones. In an entry dated November 14, 1952, after receiving a letter from Norton, who would have been hospitalized for several months at the time, she wrote:

> All right, this is it. For the first time (since I heard about Dick) I have broken down and cried, and talked, and cried and talked again. I felt the mask crumple, the great poisonous store of corrosive ashes begin to spew out of my mouth. I have been needing, more than anything, to talk to somebody, to spill out all the tight, jealous, envious, apprehensive neurotic tensions in me....
>
> All right, tonight, after good pizza, Chianti, hot coffee and laughter, I went upstairs to the green, white and red room which is light, and vitality and Marcia. There, on the bed, she touched the soft spot, the one vulnerable spot in the hard, frozen, acrid little core in me, and I could cry....
>
> And Dick is recriminating himself, readjusting, trying to grow, too. And not living in the luxurious erotic Garden of Eden I imagined, either.[1]

Months passed, during which Norton's health improved, but not as rapidly or substantially as hoped (he was destined to spend two years in Saranac Lake), and on January 10, 1953, following her winter vacation visit to Saranac Lake, Plath wrote:

> Dick and I are doomed to *compete* always and never cooperate.... I feel he wants to prove his virile dominance.... With him,...I never felt that I was *feminine*. Seeing him after two months, I no longer felt the desire flame up in me. I didn't particularly want him to touch me. For one thing, since he can't kiss me at all, I have the feeling (purely mental) that his mouth is a source of poisonous tuberculosis germs, and, therefore, unclean. I am, therefore, physically aloof.

Introspective, soul- and identity-searching, self-oriented, Plath's diary entries surrounding the time of Norton's illness deal with him only in the context of the inner tumult of their relationship. As for the tuberculosis that had isolated him, separated them, for her it exists, a barrier, perhaps—she cannot kiss him (and presumably wore a gown and mask during her visits)—but of little note and of little concern. The barrier, she believes, is in her mind and in her feelings toward Dick, more than in fact. For Sylvia Plath, a bright, articulate college student from a middle-class American family and a budding poetic genius, tuberculosis is not a dread disease. It is an annoyance, little known and poorly understood by her, but not a threat.

In 1963, writing under the pen name Victoria Lucas, Plath published a novel titled *The Bell Jar* in England; it was republished under her name in the United States in 1971.[2] This novel is widely considered to be autobiographical. The protagonist and narrator, Esther Greenwood, represents Sylvia; her boyfriend, Buddy Willard, represents Dick Norton. While much of the book probably portrays events in Plath's life, it is a mistake to read it as a literal autobiography, for some of the events described are certainly fictional. In the novel, Buddy, a medical student, develops tuberculosis, just as Norton did in life. Esther receives a phone call at her college dormitory.

> It was Buddy all right. He told me that the annual fall chest X-ray showed he had caught TB and he was going off...to a TB place in the Adirondacks.... Would I please try to write to him at least once a week and come to visit him at this TB place in my Christmas vacation?...
>
> I told Buddy how sorry I was about the TB and promised to write, but when I hung up I didn't feel one bit sorry. I only felt a wonderful relief....
>
> I thought the TB might just be a punishment for...feeling so superior to people. And I thought how convenient it would be now I didn't have to announce to everybody at college I had broken off with Buddy and start the boring business of blind dates all over again.
>
> I simply told everyone that Buddy had TB and we were practically engaged, and when I stayed in to study on Saturday nights they were extremely kind to me because they thought I was so brave, working the way I did just to hide a broken heart.[3]

Not a dread disease. Tuberculosis for Sylvia Plath was a convenience! Not a special or out-of-the ordinary affliction in her mind. Something that had happened and, for Esther/Sylvia, a convenient event. There was no particular need to be concerned about Buddy's/Dick's ultimate fate. Later in the novel, Plath reveals more concern about tuberculosis. "I had very little knowledge about TB," Esther reflects, "but it seemed to me an extremely sinister disease, the way it went on invisibly." Sinister, perhaps, and infectious, but not gravely concerning. Another disease, another need to take pills. Not another cause for alarm, not another death warrant. With the advent of modern, effective chemotherapy, tuberculosis had become curable.

During the summer of 1953 Plath became increasingly depressed, and in August she attempted suicide. Following psychiatric treatment, including hospitalization and electric shock treatment, she recovered and returned to Smith. Following graduation from Smith, she went to Cambridge in England to continue her literary studies. Her relationship with Norton was over, left behind, clearly withering and ready for an ending by both parties.

At Cambridge she met Ted Hughes, whom she married on June 16, 1956. The couple was happy. They both wrote. Sylvia obtained a faculty appointment at Smith, and in 1957 they moved to Northampton, Massachusetts, the site of Smith College. Sylvia became pregnant, but miscarried. In December of 1959 the couple sailed for England, Sylvia again pregnant, where they would pursue their increasingly noted careers as writers, find friends, and become the parents of two children.

In July 1962, Sylvia Plath discovered her husband's infidelity. Angry, she left him. Her moods became increasingly labile. Depression haunted her. On February 11, 1963, she opened the gas jets in her apartment and let the escaping fumes take her life.

In 1982 the Pulitzer Prize was awarded posthumously to Sylvia Plath for *Ariel*, the collection of poems written during the last five years of her life.

CHAPTER 14

ESSAYIST

SUSAN SONTAG, 1933–2004

—*Indifference*—

Modern disease metaphors are all cheap shots.
—*Susan Sontag,* Illness as Metaphor

SUSAN SONTAG's extended essay, *Illness as Metaphor*, is a thought-provoking, beautifully crafted examination of nineteenth-century attitudes towards tuberculosis and modern attitudes towards cancer. They are, she persuasively argues, much the same. These attitudes—metaphors, as she terms them—are important to understand, because illness should not be viewed as a metaphor. "The most truthful way of regarding illness—and the healthiest way of being ill—is one most purified of, most resistant to, metaphoric thinking" writes Sontag. "Yet it is hardly possibly to take up one's residence in the kingdom of the ill unprejudiced by the lurid metaphors with which it has been landscaped."[1]

Susan Sontag was born in New York in 1933, but was placed in the care of her grandparents in Los Angeles when her mother moved to China to join her husband, Susan's father, a fur trader. He died five years later of pulmonary tuberculosis, a diagnosis that Susan's mother hid from her for many years. When Susan was twelve, her mother remarried and moved with her and her sister to Tucson, Arizona, the home of her stepfather. Susan adopted the surname of her stepfather, Sontag.

A precocious student, Sontag graduated from high school and entered the University of Chicago in 1948 at age fifteen. Two years later she met Philip Rieff, a sociology instructor, whom she married only ten days after meeting him. She soon became pregnant and had her only child, a son, David Rieff, who later became a writer, her biographer, and her editor at Farrar, Straus and Giroux. She graduated from the University of Chicago in 1951, and moved to Harvard with her husband, who had secured a faculty position at nearby Brandeis University. At Harvard she earned master's degrees in both literature and philosophy and enrolled in a doctoral program. In 1957 she won a fellowship to study at St. Anne's College in Oxford; at the same time Rieff accepted a fellowship to study at Stanford University in California. Sontag later transferred from Oxford to the University of Paris. Mastering French easily, she came to love Paris, and in later years she spent much time there. She divorced her husband in 1959 and, penniless, moved to New York City. She quickly found teaching positions at City College of New York, Sarah Lawrence College, and Columbia University. She also found success as a writer.

Sontag's career blossomed. She earned a distinguished reputation as a film and photography critic. Her writing won awards. As her life progressed, she became a doyenne of "belles artes"; in an earlier era, she would have hosted a popular salon. Her circle of friends included most of the literary stars of the age and many liberal activists. She was an advocate of avant-garde positions. She was a feminist and a human rights activist. She was outspoken in opposition to the Vietnam War.

In October 1975, Susan Sontag, age forty-two, underwent a radical mastectomy for an invasive breast cancer. The procedure, then thought to be the optimum treatment for her type of cancer, was both disfiguring and defeminizing. Even with the surgery, she was told, her outlook was poor. She dug into medical literature and discovered that chemotherapy drugs not approved by the Food and Drug Administration and hence not available in America were being used to treat breast cancer in Europe. She went to Paris, and there received weekly chemotherapy treatments for the next two and one-half years. It was during this time that she wrote *Illness as Metaphor.*

Sontag recovered her health and resumed her active life. She remained well for more than two decades. In 1998, however, her cancer recurred. More chemotherapy followed. So also did pain and anguish. The cancer took her life on December 28, 2004.

Illness as Metaphor is one of Sontag's best known works. Before examining its messages, it is worth remembering that her father died of tuberculosis, although she could scarcely have known him. His diagnosis was hidden from her, perhaps considered shameful. More importantly, one should be cognizant of the fact that Sontag, herself, was living with cancer—breast cancer, in her case—as she worked on the essay.

Sontag's thesis in *Illness as Metaphor* is that the romanticism, shame, and other attributes associated with tuberculosis in the nineteenth century have, with better understanding of that disease, been transferred to cancer in modern times. Indeed much of the earlier thinking about tuberculosis was conditioned by the fact that its cause was not known before Koch's discovery of the tubercle bacillus.

> The notion that a disease can be explained only by a variety of [unknown] causes is precisely characteristic of thinking about diseases whose causation is not understood.

Such thinking serves those now afflicted with devastating disease no better than it did Victorian era victims. In Sontag's view, that time was a romantic one, and "TB was a disease in the service of a romantic view of the world." The romanticism associated with tuberculosis came at a price.

> What once made TB seem so interesting—or, as it was usually put, romantic—also made it a curse and a source of special dread.... TB was understood as a disease that isolates one from the community. However steep its incidence in a population, TB—like cancer today—always seemed to be a mysterious disease of individuals, a deadly arrow that could strike anyone, that singled out its victims one by one.

Sontag describes the metaphors associated with tuberculosis, that is, the then current attitudes towards it, in considerable detail.

> TB...[has] been used to express not only...crude fantasies about contamination but also fairly complex feelings about strength and weakness, and about energy. For more than a century and a half, tuberculosis provided a metaphoric equivalent for delicacy, sensitivity, sadness, powerlessness.... TB was an ambivalent metaphor, both a scourge and an emblem of refinement.

Sontag's essay says much about nineteenth-century attitudes towards tuberculosis and other plagues of earlier times, but it says little about modern attitudes towards this disease. Rather, Sontag emphasizes that earlier attitudes towards tuberculosis have now shifted to other diseases, including cancer, which had afflicted her.

> In the twentieth century the cluster of metaphors and attitudes formerly attached to TB split up and are parceled out to two diseases. Some features of TB go to insanity: the notion of the sufferer as a hectic, reckless creature of passionate extremes, someone too sensitive to bear the horrors of the vulgar, everyday world. Other features of TB go to cancer—the agonies that can't be romanticized. Not TB but insanity is the current vehicle of our secular myth of self-transcendence. The romantic view is that illness exacerbates consciousness. Once that illness was TB; now it is insanity that is thought to bring consciousness to a state of paroxysmic enlightenment. The romanticizing of madness reflects in the most vehement way the contemporary prestige of irrational or rude (spontaneous) behavior (acting-out), of that very passionateness whose repression was once imagined to cause TB, and is now thought to cause cancer.

In reading Sontag's work, one is struck by the paucity of attention given to current perceptions of tuberculosis. In an earlier century, she notes, tuberculosis was surrounded by fear. Attitudes of despair often cloaked in romanticism were once common and dominated public perceptions of the disease. Not so, however, for Sontag as she puts her reactions to paper in a more modern time. This disease is no longer of interest. It is simply another annoyance. Today, she argues, "there is no disgrace, nothing of the taboo that once surrounded people afflicted with TB." Sontag's perceptions of tuberculosis are most clearly expressed by what she did not write. Tuberculosis has become unimportant.

PART V

TSUNAMI ALERT

—The Unending Quest—

CHAPTER 15

CODA

1981–?

Whereof what's past is prologue, what to come
In yours and my discharge.
—*William Shakespeare,* The Tempest, *Act II, Scene 1*

MEDICAL SCIENCE is not static. The quest to conquer tuberculosis is an ongoing one. While the records of history provide many insights into the battle against tuberculosis, there are yet more insights to be gained, and there is yet more history to be written. Most would agree that the major challenges for tuberculosis control today and in the foreseeable future are presented by the coincident prevalence of AIDS (acquired immunodeficiency syndrome) and tuberculosis, the emergence of multidrug-resistant tubercle bacilli, and the need for an effective vaccine to protect against the disease.

On June 5, 1981 the United States Public Health Service Centers for Disease Control published in its *Morbidity and Mortality Weekly Report* (*MMWR*) a description of five cases of *Pneumocystis carinii* (*Pneumocystis jiroveci*) pneumonia among five previously healthy men in Los Angeles.[1] This rare pneumonia had generally been seen previously only in persons undergoing cancer chemotherapy or otherwise severely immunocompromised. All five men in this first description of what soon became known as AIDS were described as "homosexuals." Eighteen months later, the new syndrome was reported in ten previously healthy heterosexual men who had immigrated to the United States from Haiti, six of whom had tuberculosis.[2] At about the same time as these reports of disease in Americans and Haitians, "slim disease" was noted in rural Central Africa.[3] In 1983 the catalog of persons susceptible to the AIDS virus was extended to patients with hemophilia being supported with transfused antihemophilic factor obtained from donated blood.[4]

It was not long before it was recognized that tuberculosis is a major problem for patients with AIDS. Doctors Gnana Sunderam, Lee Reichman, and their coworkers in New Jersey noted that many of their tuberculosis patients who also had AIDS presented with unusual clinical pictures.[5] They suggested that tuberculosis should be considered as one of the defining infections for the AIDS syndrome. Dr. Arthur Pitchenick and his colleagues in Florida noted that tuberculosis and AIDS were occurring concomitantly in Haitian immigrants whom they saw in their clinic.[6] Throughout Sub-Saharan Africa it soon became apparent that tuberculosis was the leading infection occurring in immunosuppressed AIDS patients and the cause of death in most AIDS sufferers. In Kampala, Uganda, two-thirds of tuberculosis patients were found to suffer from AIDS.[7] In Abidjan, Côte d'Ivoire, the figure was 44 percent.[8]

AIDS and tuberculosis became known as "the cursed duet." The AIDS virus attacks the lymphocytic cells primarily responsible for the body's defense against tubercle bacilli. AIDS dramatically increases susceptibility to tuberculosis.

It is easy to note that tuberculosis and AIDS go hand in hand, and that it is in Sub-Saharan Africa that the convergence of these two killers is at its worst. More money to combat AIDS and more money to treat and control tuberculosis will help. But even more is needed—more knowledge of the fundamental defects in immunity that fan the flames of these often smoldering infections into deadly disease. Immunologists and immunopathologists today are rising to this challenge, assisted by epidemiologists who chart the firestorm track. They work in laboratories in London, Bethesda, and Cleveland, and also Johannesburg, Nairobi, and Kampala.

In 1991 a young physician moved to Cleveland after finishing specialty training in Cincinnati, Ohio. While an intern in 1984, the new medical school graduate had developed tuberculosis and been treated with a usually curative three-drug regimen of isoniazid, rifampin, and ethambutol. Two years later, a chest X-ray film showed progression, and the young doctor received another course of treatment with the same drugs. As part of a hospital credentialing procedure shortly after arrival in Cleveland, a chest radiograph was taken. It showed progression of the tuberculosis, and a CT scan demonstrated a new tuberculous cavity. With a presumptive diagnosis of multidrug-resistant (MDR) tuberculosis—later confirmed in the laboratory—the doctor was treated with second-line drugs and surgical resection of the diseased lung lobe. He remained well thereafter.

Strain W *Mycobacterium tuberculosis* probably originated in China (it has become known as the Beijing strain). Over time it developed resistance to isoniazid, rifampin, and streptomycin, and this now multidrug-resistant strain was given the designation W-12.[9] The first documented case of W-12 disease was the doctor recognized in Cleveland in 1991 who had been infected in Cincinnati in 1984. In 1992 strain W-12 reached New York City and then the New York State prison system.[10] It spread rapidly and was deadly in those infected with AIDS virus and in a prison guard who was immunosuppressed while receiving chemotherapy for cancer. It produced indolent disease in immunologically normal persons, just as it did for many years in the physician infected in Cincinnati. Subsequently it has continued to spread, circling the globe.

Much of the multidrug-resistant tuberculosis burden is spawned by interrupted therapy. In Russian prisons a failure of drug supply chains created the problem. The Russian penal system houses approximately one million prisoners. About 300,000 are released to return to society each year. About ten percent of Russian prisoners have active tuberculosis, and one-third of them have multidrug-resistant disease—10,000 persons with MDR tuberculosis returned to Russian communities each year. Writing about this situation, tuberculosis expert Dr. Lee Reichman called it a "time bomb."[11] In Russian prisons the problem did not lie with the prisoners nor their doctors. Rather, the administrative system failed to provide a continuous supply of drugs. Drug resistance is fostered by interrupted therapy.

In rural Sub-Saharan Africa a seemingly insurmountable complex of logistical, economic, and cultural impediments stymied efforts to provide uninterrupted successful drug treatment. Yet, under daunting circumstances, dedicated health care providers have shown that these barriers can be overcome. However, at present, there is a limited arsenal of bactericidal drugs for the treatment and retreatment of drug-resistant tuberculosis.

In 2006 South African tuberculosis scientists reported an outbreak of tuberculosis in miners in Kwazulu-Natal due to a strain of *M. tuberculosis* resistant to five drugs, including both isoniazid and rifampin.[12] Fifty-three men were afflicted. They all were also infected with the AIDS virus. All died, with an average survival time after diagnosis of only sixteen days. The South Africans termed this disease extensively drug-resistant (XDR). Since then, XDR tuberculosis has been recognized throughout the world; it now accounts for about one percent of tubercle bacilli studied in national reference laboratories.[13] This is probably a biased incidence figure, for troublesome cases are those most likely to have their cultures studied in national reference laboratories. Nonetheless, XDR tuberculosis is a matter of global concern.

Microbiologists and molecular biologists have unraveled the genetic codes of many strains of tubercle bacilli. Their work will point the way to targets in the organism that pharmacologists and biochemists can pursue in designing new drugs. What will prevent tubercle bacilli from developing resistance to each newly developed drug? Only the work of dedicated care givers who establish treatment programs that ensure uninterrupted patient compliance.

—

Over the course of history vaccines have provided the most effective means of preventing infectious diseases. A vaccine for tuberculosis exists (BCG). The story of this vaccine is one of false starts and discouraging failures.[14] Yet a vaccine should be possible. As new knowledge of the antigens of mycobacteria emerges from the laboratories of microbiologists, immunochemists, and molecular geneticists, new vaccine targets will become evident. The challenges of evaluating candidate vaccines against tuberculosis in large population studies are awesome. Surrogate markers of immunity must be found, and epidemiological tools for early evaluation of effectiveness are needed.

—

The challenges are not limited to medical clinics of tuberculosis doctors and the benches of laboratory scientists. Behavioral, cultural, and organizational issues surround the conduct of tuberculosis control efforts in many venues. Social and political scientists must bring their disciplines and skills to the front ranks of tuberculosis control programs.

There is little doubt that progress is being made in the continuing quest to conquer tuberculosis. Much is happening. And there is every reason to hope that there will be more and more progress. The quest seems unending, but advances are being made, and with them there can be renewed hope. The trail forward is being blazed.

NOTES

CHAPTER 1. CHANGE, PAGES 7–29

1. Charles Dickens, *Nicholas Nickleby* (New York, NY: Barnes & Noble Classics, 2005).
2. *Ibid.*
3. James Clark, *A Treatise on Pulmonary Consumption; Comprehending an Inquiry into the Causes, Nature, Prevention, and Treatment of Tuberculous and Scrofulous Diseases in General* (Philadelphia, PA: Carey, Lea, and Blanchard, 1835).
4. *Ibid.*
5. *Ibid.*
6. Jean-Antoine Villemin, *Étude Sur la Tuberculose* (Paris: Baillère, 1868). Translated in Ralph H. Major, *Classic Descriptions of Disease,* 3rd ed. (Springfield, IL: Charles C. Thomas, 1945).
7. S. Adolphus Knopf, "The centenary of Brehmer's birth," *American Review of Tuberculosis* 14 (1926): 207-210.
8. Hugh M. Kinghorn, "Brehmer and Dettweiler. A review of their methods of treatment of pulmonary tuberculosis," *American Review of Tuberculosis* 5 (1922): 950-972.
9. Editorial, *British Journal of Tuberculosis* 1 (1907): 1-4.
10. Quoted in Ray Robinson, *Matty. An American Hero. Christy Mathewson of the New York Giants* (New York, NY: Oxford University Press, 1993).
11. Quoted in Thomas D. Brock, *Robert Koch: A life in medicine and bacteriology* (New York: Springer-Verlag, 1988).
12. J. Burns Amberson Jr., B.T. McMahon, and Max Pinner, "A clinical trial of sanocrysin in pulmonary tuberculosis," *American Review of Tuberculosis* 24 (1931): 401-434.
13. Frederick Bernheim, "The effect of salicylate on the oxygen uptake of the tubercle bacillus," *Science* 92 (1940): 204.
14. Irving J. Selikoff, Edward H. Robitzek, and George G. Ornstein, "Treatment of pulmonary tuberculosis with hydrazide derivatives of isonicotinic acid," *Journal of the American Medical Association* 150 (1952): 973-980.

15. Thomas M. Daniel, "Rifampin—a major new chemotherapeutic agent for the treatment of tuberculosis," *New England Journal of Medicine* 280 (1969): 615-616.

CHAPTER 2. ROMANTIC POET, PAGES 33–43

1. John Keats to John Hamilton Reynolds, Sunday, 3 May 1818. Maurice Buxton Forman, ed., *The Letters of John Keats. Second Edition* (New York, NY: Oxford University Press, 1935).
2. John Keats, "Ode on a Grecian Urn," Howard Foster Lowry and Willard Thorp, eds., *An Anthology of English Poetry* (New York, NY: Oxford University Press, 1935).
3. Charles Armitage Brown, *Life of John Keats.* Dorothy Hyde Bodurtha and Willard Bissell Pope, eds. (London: Oxford University Press, 1937).
4. Walter A. Wells, *A Doctor's Life of Keats* (New York: Vantage Press, 1959).
5. Percy Bysshe Shelley to John Keats, 27 July 1827. Walter A. Wells, Op. cit.
6. John Keats to Fanny Brawne, August 1820. Maurice Buxton Forman, *Op. cit.*
7. John Keats to John Taylor, Monday, 14 August, 1820. Maurice Buxton Forman, *Op. cit.*
8. John Keats to Charles Brown, August 1820. Maurice Buxton Forman, *Op. cit.*
9. John Keats, "Sonnet. Bright Star," Howard Foster Lowry and Willard Thorp, eds., *Op. cit.*
10. John Keats, "Ode to a Nightingale," Howard Foster Lowry and Willard Thorp, eds. *Op. cit.*
11. John Keats to Charles Brown, Wednesday, 1 November 1820. Maurice Buxton Forman. *Op. cit.*

CHAPTER 3. THE CONSUMPTIVE BRONTËS, PAGES 44–45

1. John Bunyon, *The Life and Death of Mr. Badman* (New York, NY: R. H. Russell, 1900.)
2. Elizabeth C. Gaskell, *The Life of Charlotte Brontë, Author of "Jane Eyre," "Shirley," "Vilette," &c* (New York, NY: D. Appleton and Company, 1858).
3. A. Mary F. Robinson, *Emily Brontë* (London: Wyman and Sons, Limited, 1883).

4. Emily Brontë, *Wuthering Heights* (New York, NY: Barnes & Noble Classics, 2004). Originally published in 1847 under the pseudonym Ellis Bell. Subsequent quotations are from this edition.
5. Charlotte Brontë to Ellen Nussey, October 1848. Elizabeth C. Gaskell, *Op. cit.*
6. Charlotte Brontë to Ellen Nussey, 1848. Muriel Spark, ed., *The Letters of the Brontës: A Selection* (Norman, OK: University of Oklahoma Press, 1954).
7. Charlotte Brontë to Ellen Nussey, 25 November, 1848. Elizabeth C. Gaskell, *Op. cit.*
8. Charlotte Brontë to Ellen Nussey, 18 December, 1848. Muriel Spark, *Op. cit.*
9. Currer Bell (Charlotte Brontë), "Biographical Notice of Ellis and Acton Bell," preface to the 1850 edition of *Wuthering Heights*. Reprinted in Emily Brontë, *Wuthering Heights* (New York, NY: Barnes & Noble Classics, 2004).
10. Charlotte Brontë to Ellen Nussey, 23 December 1848. Muriel Spark, *Op. cit.*
11. Charlotte Brontë to William Smith Williams, 1848. Rebecca Fraser, *The Brontës: Charlotte Brontë and Her Family* (Crown Publishers, Inc., New York, NY, 1988).
12. Charlotte Brontë to Ellen Nussey, 15 January 1849. Muriel Spark, *Op. cit.*
13. Anne Brontë to Ellen Nussey, 15 April 1849. Muriel Spark, *Op. cit.*
14. Charlotte Brontë to William Smith Williams, 11 June 1849. Muriel Spark, *Op. cit.*
15. Anne Brontë, *The Tenant of Wildfell Hall* (Oxford: Oxford University Press, 1992). Originally published in 1848 under the pseudonym Acton Bell.
16. Charlotte Brontë, *Jane Eyre* (New York, NY: Barnes & Noble Classics, 2003). Originally published in 1847 under the pseudonym Currer Bell.
17. Charlotte Brontë to Laetitia Wheelwright, 15 February 1855. Elizabeth C. Gaskell, *Op. cit.*
18. Charlotte Brontë to Ellen Nussey, March 1855. Winifred Gérin, *Charlotte Brontë: The Evolution of a Genius* (Oxford; The Clarendon Press, 1967).

CHAPTER 4. NATURALIST, PAGES 56–62

1. Henry David Thoreau to Charles Wyatt Rice, 5 August 1836. Walter Harding and Carl Bode, *The Correspondence of Henry David Thoreau* (New York, NY: New York University Press, 1958).
2. Walter Harding, *The Days of Henry Thoreau* (New York, NY: Alfred A. Knopf, 1965).
3. Henry David Thoreau to Harrison G. O. Blake, 27 June 1855. Walter Harding and Carl Bode, *Op. cit.*
4. *Down at the Lake. A Historical Portrait of Linden Hills and the Lake Harriet District* (Minneapolis, MN: Linden Hills History Study Group, 2002).
5. Henry David Thoreau to Messrs. Editors, February 11, 1862. Walter Harding and Carl Bode, *Op. cit.*
6. Linck C. Johnson, *Thoreau's Complex Weave: The Writing of A Week on the Concord and Merrimack Rivers with the Text of the First Draft* (Charlottesville, VA: University Press of Virginia, 1986).
7. Henry David Thoreau to Harrison G. O. Blake, 6 December 1856. Walter Harding and Carl Bode, *Op. cit.*

CHAPTER 5. VOICE OF THE SOUTH, PAGES 63–69

1. William Hayes Ward, *Memorial*, in Sidney Lanier, *Poems of Sidney Lanier, Edited by His Wife* (New York, NY: Charles Scribner's Sons, 1929). Subsequent quotations from Lanier's letters are from the same source.
2. Sidney Lanier, *Poems of Sidney Lanier, Edited by His Wife, Op. cit.* Subsequent quotations from Lanier's poems are from this source.
3. Edd Winfield Parks, *Sidney Lanier: The Man, the Poet, The Critic* (Athens, GA: University of Georgia press, 1968).
4. Mary Day Lanier in William Hayes Ward, *Op. cit.*

CHAPTER 6. DEMI-MONDE, PAGES 70–77

1. Alexandre Dumas *fils* to Marie Duplessis. Virginia Rounding, *Grandes Horizontales. The Lives and Legends of Marie Duplessis, Cora Pearl, La Païva and La Présidente* (New York, NY: Bloomsbury, 2003).
2. Alexandre Dumas *fils*, *La Dame aux camélias: Camille: The Authorized Translation into English by Edmond Gosse with an Introduction by André Maurois, a Prefatory Letter from the Author and A Memoir*

of Marie Duplessis by Jules Janin (New York, NY: The Heritage Press, 1955).

3. Alexandre Dumas *fils*, *Camille: The Lady of Camellias,* translated by Henriette Metcalf (New York, NY: Samuel French, Inc., 1959). Subsequent quotations are from this source.
4. *Ibid.*
5. Giuseppe Verdi, *La Traviata.* Libretto by Francesco Maria Piave (New York, NY: BMG Music, 1991). Subsequent quotations from *La Traviata* are from this source.
6. Alexandre Dumas *fils*, 1959, *Op. cit.*
7. *Ibid.*
8. Roger Ingpen and Walter E. Peck, eds., *The Complete Works of Percy Bysshe Shelley: Volume III: Poems* (New York, NY: Gordian Press, 1965).
9. Alexandre Dumas *fils*, 1959. *Op. cit.*
10. *Ibid.*

CHAPTER 7. BOHEMIA, PAGES 78–83

1. Henri Murger, *The Bohemians of the Latin Quarter (Scènes de la vie de bohème)* (London: Gibbings & Company, Limited, 1895). Henry Mürger, *Vie de bohème,* translation by Norman Cameron (London: Folio Society, 1960).
2. Arthur Moss and Evalyn Marvel, *The Legend of the Latin Quarter; Henry Mürger and the Birth of Bohemia* (New York, NY: The Beechhurst Press, 1946). Mürger's play is not available in English translation. The action is summarized by Moss and Marvel.
3. Henry Mürger, 1960. *Op cit.*
4. *Ibid.*

CHAPTER 8. MAGIC MOUNTAIN, PAGES 87–100

1. Thomas Mann, "The Making of *The Magic Mountain,*" afterword in the Vintage International edition of Thomas Mann, *The Magic Mountain (Der Zauberberg),* translated from the German by H.T. Lowe-Porter (New York, NY: Vintage International, 1992). A note indicates that Mann's essay was first published in *The Atlantic* in January 1953.
2. *Ibid.*

3. Thomas Mann, *The Magic Mountain (Der Zauberberg),* translated from the German by H.T. Lowe-Porter (New York, NY: Vintage International, 1992). Other quotes from this work are from the same edition.

4. Thomas Mann, *A Sketch of My Life*. Hans Bürgin and Hans-Otto Mayer. *Thomas Mann: A Chronicle of His Life*. English Translation by Eugene Dobson (Tuscaloosa, Alabama: University of Alabama Press, 1965).

CHAPTER 9. STORY TELLER, PAGES 101–114

1. David Garnett to Jeffrey Meyers, 24 November 1975. Jeffrey Meyers, *Katherine Mansfield. A Biography* (New York, NY: New Directions, 1980).
2. Katherine Mansfield, *Journal of Katherine Mansfield,* edited by J. Middleton Murry (New York, NY: Alfred A. Knopf, 1959).
3. *Ibid.*
4. Katherine Mansfield, *The Collected Letters of Katherine Mansfield. Volume Four. 1920-1921*, Appendix, edited by Vincent O'Sullivan and Margaret Scott (Oxford: Clarendon Press, 1996).
5. Katherine Mansfield, *Letters to John Middleton Murry: 1913-1922,* edited by John Middleton Murry (New York, NY: Alfred A. Knopf, 1951).
6. *Ibid.*
7. Katherine Mansfield, *Journal of Katherine Mansfield,* edited by J. Middleton Murry. *Op. cit.*
8. *Ibid.*
9. *Ibid.*
10. Katherine Mansfield, *Letters to John Middleton Murry: 1913-1922,* edited by John Middleton Murry. *Op. cit.* Subsequent quotations from her letters to Murry are from the same source.
11. Katherine Mansfield, "The Fly." *The Short Stories of Katherine Mansfield* (New York, NY: Alfred A. Knopf, 1937).

CHAPTER 10. ARISTOCRAT, PAGES 115–121

1. W. Somerset Maugham, "Sanatorium." *The Complete Short Stories of W. Somerset Maugham: II: The World Over* (Garden City, NY: Doubleday & Company, Inc., 1952). All subsequent excerpts and quotations are from this edition.

CHAPTER 11. CHAMPION, PAGES 122–130

1. Alice Marble with Dale Leatherman, *Courting Danger* (New York, NY: St. Martin's Press, 1991). Subsequent quotations from this autobiography are from the same edition.
2. Francis Marion Pottenger, *Tuberculosis: A Discussion of Phthisiogenesis, Immunology, Pathologic Physiology, Diagnosis, and Treatment* (St. Louis, MO: The C.V. Mosby Company, 1948).
3. *Ibid.*

CHAPTER 12. THE RACK, PAGES 131–144

1. A.E. Ellis, *The Rack* (Boston, MA: Little, Brown and Company, 1958).
2. *Ibid.* Additional quotations from this work are from the same edition.
3. Katherine Mansfield, "The Fly." *The Short Stories of Katherine Mansfield* (New York, NY: Alfred A. Knopf, 1937).
4. This quotation is from the end of the last scene of William Shakespeare, *King Lear.*

CHAPTER 13. MODERN POET, PAGES 147–151

1. Karen V. Kukil, ed., *The Unabridged Journals of Sylvia Plath: 1950-1962: Transcribed from the Original Manuscripts at Smith College* (New York, NY: Anchor Books, 2000). Subsequent quotations from her diary are from this source.
2. Sylvia Plath, *The Bell Jar* (New York, NY: Harper & Row Publishers, 1971).
3. *Ibid.*

CHAPTER 14. ESSAYIST, PAGES 152–156

1. Susan Sontag, *Illness as Metaphor* (New York, NY: Farrar, Straus and Giroux, 1978). Subsequent quotations are from this edition.

CHAPTER 15. CODA, PAGES 159–163

1. Centers for Disease Control, "Pneumocystis pneumonia—Los Angeles," *Morbidity and Mortality Weekly Report* 30 (1981): 250-252.
2. Jeffrey Vieira, Elliot Frank, Thomas J. Spira and Sheldon H. Landesman, "Acquired Immune Deficiency in Haitians. Opportunistic Infections in Previously Healthy Haitian Immigrants," *New England Journal of Medicine* 308 (1983): 125-129.

3. D. Serwadda, R.D. Mugerwa, N.K. Sewankambo, A. Lwegaba, J.W. Carswell, G.B. Kirya, A.C. Bayley, R.G. Downing, R.S. Tedder, S.A. Clayden, A.G. Dalgleish, "Slim Disease: A New Disease in Uganda and Its Association with HTLV-III Infection," *Lancet* 2 (1985): 849-852.

4. Michael M. Lederman, Oscar D. Ratnoff, James J. Scillian, Paul K. Jones and Bernice Schacter, "Impaired Cell-Mediated Immunity in Patients with Classic Hemophilia," *New England Journal of Medicine* 308 (1983): 79-83.

5. Gnana Sunderam, Reynard J. McDonald, Theodore Maniatis, James Oleske, Rajendra Kapila and Lee B. Reichman, "Tuberculosis as a Manifestation of the Acquired Immunodeficiency Syndrome (AIDS)," *JAMA* 256 (1986): 362-366.

6. Arthur E. Pitchenik, Clifford Cole, Bertrand W. Russell, Margaret A. Fischl, Thomas J. Spira and Dixie E. Snider, Jr., "Tuberculosis, Atypical Mycobacteriosis, and the Acquired Immunodeficiency Syndrome Among Haitian and Non-Haitian Patients in South Florida," *Annals of Internal Medicine* 101 (1984): 641-645. Arthur E. Pitchenik, Janice Burr, Manuel Suarez, Deborah Fertel, Gerardo Gonzalez and Carlos Moas, "Human T-Cell Lymphotropic Virus-III (HTLV-III) Seropositivity and Related Disease Among 71 Consecutive Patients in Whom Tuberculosis Was Diagnosed: A Prospective Study," *American Review of Respiratory Disease* 135: (1987): 875-879.

7. Peter P. Eriki, Alphonse Okwera, Tom Aisu, Anne B. Morrissey, Jerrold J. Ellner and Thomas M. Daniel, "The Influence of Human Immunodeficiency Virus (HIV) on Tuberculosis in Kampala, Uganda," *American Review of Respiratory Disease* 143 (1991): 185-187.

8. S.B. Richards, M.E. St. Louis, P. Nieburg, I.M. Coulibaly, D. Coulibaly, L. Abouya, H. D. Gayle and K.M. DeCock, "Impact of the HIV Epidemic on Trends in Tuberculosis in Abidjan, Côte d'Ivoire," *Tubercle and Lung Disease* 76 (1995): 11-16.

9. Pablo J. Bifani, Bonnie B. Plikaytis, Vivek Kapur, Kathryn Stockbauer, Xi Pan, Michael L. Lutfey, Soraya L. Moghazeh, William Eisner, Thomas M. Daniel, Mark H. Kaplan, Jack T. Crawford, James M. Musser and Barry N. Kreiswirth, "Origin and Interstate Spread of a New York City Multidrug-Resistant *Mycobacterium tuberculosis* Clone Family," *JAMA* 275 (1996): 452-457.

10. Sarah E. Valway, Robert B. Greifinger, Mark Papania, James O. Kilburn, Charles Woodley, George T. DiFerdinando and Samuel W.

Dooley, "Multidrug-Resistant Tuberculosis in the New York State Prison System," *Journal of Infectious Diseases* 170 (1994): 151-156.

11. Lee B. Reichman with Janice Hopkins Tanne, *Timebomb: The Global Epidemic of Multi-Drug-Resistant Tuberculosis* (New York, NY. McGraw-Hill, 2002).
12. Jon Cohen, "Extensively Drug-Resistant TB Gets Foothold in South Africa," *Science* 313 (2006): 1554.
13. Centers for Disease Control and Prevention, "Plan to Combat Extensively Drug-Resistant Tuberculosis: Recommendations of the Federal Tuberculosis Task Force," *MMWR* 58, RR-3 (2009): 1-43.
14. Paul E.M. Fine, "The BCG story: Lessons from the Past and Implications for the Future," *Reviews of Infectious Disease* 11 Suppl. (1989): S353-S359.